owning your
menopause

FITTER,
CALMER,
STRONGER
in 30 days

T0301224

KATE ROWE-HAM

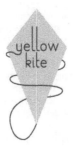

yellow
kite

First published in Great Britain in 2023 by Yellow Kite
An imprint of Hodder & Stoughton
An Hachette UK company

5

Copyright © Kate Rowe-Ham 2023

The right of Kate Rowe-Ham to be identified as the Author
of the Work has been asserted by her in accordance with
the Copyright, Designs and Patents Act 1988.

Illustrations © WorkoutLabs, LLC. (reproduced with their
permission) except pages 74, 224 and 245 © shutterstock.com

A CIP catalogue record for this title is available from the British Library

*The information in this book is not intended to replace or conflict with the advice
given to you by your doctor or other health professional. All matters regarding
your health should be discussed with your doctor. If you have any health
concerns regarding the fitness plan, we recommend that you consult with your
doctor before you embark on it. The author and publisher disclaim any liability
directly or indirectly from the use of the material in this book by any person.*

Kate would like to say a HUGE thank you to all the experts who gave
specific contributions in their area of expertise: Dr Naomi Potter, Thryn
Pinkham, Anna Gough, Katie Skrine and Clare Bourne. Thank you all for
your time and willingness to help. Particular thanks to Katie Skrine, who
is also the in-house nutritionist for the Owning Your Menopause app.

Trade paperback ISBN 978 1 399 72583 5
ebook ISBN 978 1 399 72584 2

Typeset in Magneta Book by Hewer Text UK Ltd, Edinburgh
Printed and bound in Great Britain by Clays Ltd, Elcograf S.p.A.

Hodder & Stoughton policy is to use papers that are natural, renewable
and recyclable products and made from wood grown in sustainable
forests. The logging and manufacturing processes are expected to
conform to the environmental regulations of the country of origin.

Yellow Kite
Hodder & Stoughton Ltd
Carmelite House
50 Victoria Embankment
London EC4Y 0DZ

www.yellowkitebooks.co.uk

CONTENTS

WHO AM I AND WHY AM I WRITING THIS BOOK?

I am Kate, a wife, a mum of three and a personal trainer (PT), who specialises in helping midlife women thrive through menopause.

I've always had an interest in exercise and enjoyed sports growing up, but in all honesty, for most of my adult life I only exercised to stay slim. However, my whole relationship with exercise and my body image has changed since qualifying as a PT and going through my own journey and experiences of perimenopause. In the process, I've learnt so much about myself, completely changed how I look at my body and have started a whole new business and community to help women going through menopause.

Back in 2018, I created an Instagram account offering free workouts for busy mums like me. Over the following 2 years, however, I started to find it harder to recover from the HIIT workouts I was doing, gradually developing more aches and pains, while my anxiety went through the roof.

I didn't know what these changes were and, as you'll see, I was remarkably unprepared when the symptoms of perimenopause hit me. Talking to others since then, I know I'm not alone. I'll talk in more detail about my own story later in the book. I know this will be different from yours, but in sharing, I hope you will see how natural this change is and that what we experience as women can be a positive thing, even if it doesn't feel that way at the time – I know it didn't for me.

It seems like the whole subject of the menopause has become

2 OWNING YOUR MENOPAUSE

much more visible in the past few years, and that's a good thing. Women no longer need to suffer debilitating symptoms in silence. There is advice from trusted voices and as the medical profession becomes better informed, there is more access to treatments to alleviate symptoms, most notably HRT.

This book was born from my absolute passion to help empower, educate and support women like me and you to know that you can get your life back on track, even if, in this instant, you feel like you can't.

Menopause is a time of change – a chance to re-evaluate all sorts of things. On a physical level, it can be an opportunity to get to know your body better. You can carry on as you were before – which is what I did to start with – or you can use it as a catalyst for change. If you inform yourself about the physical changes you're going through, you will be better attuned to your body and can experiment with lifestyle changes like moving more or changing what you eat.

Some of you will resonate with the idea that exercise has purely an aesthetic benefit – it's there to make us look better. Others of you will have had the fortune of never having entertained this thought. Wherever you fall on that spectrum, perhaps hitting menopause will prompt you to try to do things a little differently.

My experience has led me to rethink what I knew about exercise and eating well. I have learnt to accept my body, and I feel fitter, calmer, stronger and more energised. While trying to manage the physical symptoms of my menopause, I've gained a far more profound understanding of myself, which has transformed and deepened my relationships with others, leading to a greater sense of community.

If this all sounds a bit Pollyanna-ish now, I ask you to be patient. If someone had told me that menopause was a positive thing when I was in the grip of it a few years ago, I would have said, 'Yeah, right!' or something much ruder, but this book aims to show that it can be so.

I hope to give you the confidence to manage your symptoms and understand that you don't need to be afraid of what you are experiencing. It will take time and energy, but if you follow some of the ideas and advice you are about to get on the importance of incorporating movement, weights and sensible eating into your lifestyle, you will be fitter, calmer and stronger in 30 days and, more importantly, for the rest of your life, regardless of your starting point.

MY PERIMENOPAUSE SO FAR

Sitting on the edge of my bed and in tears, I turn to Gerry, my husband, and say if I don't wake up, tell them it was my heart, tell them I couldn't breathe.

As always, I am woken early by my youngest and, weirdly, I am grateful. Grateful to have made it through the night.

I'm always tired. It takes me so long to go to sleep for fear of not waking up, only for my sleep to be disrupted by sweats – proper bed-wetting sweats, T-shirt-changing sweats. This constant, excruciating pain in the back of my neck and between my shoulder blades is unbearable. My GP prescribes Naproxen to no avail. On top of all these aches, pains, sweats and sleeplessness is the most frightening sense of anger. I am always angry with my kids and with my husband. And I feel detached and guilty about being unreasonable about everything. I think I must continue and keep pushing through, but deep down, I am petrified.

I can't pinpoint when I felt brave enough to call the doctor, but I knew I couldn't live like this. Unfortunately, my timing was terrible. It was March 2020 and the lockdown had begun. Unable to see the doctor in person and only having the capacity to explain my symptoms, I had very little success with my GP and I felt scared and alone. I rang my GP fortnightly for over 2 months, never speaking to the same one, going over and over my symptoms, often crying in desperation to be heard.

The upshot from these often frantic calls to my doctor was a diagnosis that I was probably overtraining, and the aches and pains I was experiencing were muscle soreness. However, I was offered no explanations for my heart palpitations, breathlessness, night sweats, anger and feelings of loneliness.

The muscle soreness came and went.

The anger came in waves.

My breathlessness and heart palpitations increased, making me more irritated, alone and invisible.

I drank more alcohol to help numb the pain and manage my anxiety.

I rang the doctor again in early July 2020 and was finally sent for several blood tests and a chest X-ray, which thankfully came back clear, but it still didn't answer how I was feeling. It was suggested at this point that I was suffering from anxiety and depression. I wasn't ashamed of this diagnosis, but I knew it wasn't that, and I felt like I had no choice but to try and diagnose myself.

I recalled hearing many of my friends talking about the menopause causing hot flashes and rage, so I started to look at the possibility that the symptoms I was experiencing might be related to my hormones in some way. However, I struggled with the distinct lack of information and the term menopause bought up images I could not relate to, with much of the data suggesting I was too young.

I began to share my experiences on Instagram and realised I wasn't alone. It was here that I had the pleasure of connecting with Dr Rebecca Lewis at Newson Health, and I did my first live Instagram chat with her in July to help others. However, it was then the penny dropped. I was perimenopausal. Following my conversations with Dr Lewis, I began tracking my feelings, symptoms, and cycle.

On 24 September 2020, my dad was diagnosed with stage IV pancreatic cancer and given months to live. I realised at this point I needed to get help to function in order to care for my dad. I took the plunge and booked an appointment with Dr Lewis. Despite receiving HRT following a diagnosis of perimenopause, I stared at the box of patches and tablets for 6 weeks, still unsure this would work. Eventually, I started and found the main difference it made was impacting my night sweats. I was a little disappointed as I had assumed that starting HRT would make me feel better and relieve all my symptoms.

At the end of December, with an exhausted body due to caring for Dad, managing my own family and drinking too much, I realised that to give myself the best chance of responding to HRT I needed to look a little closer at my lifestyle choices.

In January 2021, I committed to a Dry January. As I began to notice improvements, we went into lockdown again and I decided to remove alcohol from my life for the foreseeable future. Not only did being alcohol-free enable me to do a lot of soul-searching and give me time to reflect, but it also allowed me to realise that while one is going through perimenopause and all the extra strains and stresses that come with midlife, alcohol and diet play a fundamental role in managing many of the associated symptoms.

As I continued to research how I could thrive at this time, it became apparent that I also needed to look at how I was training. So here I am, 3 years into managing my lifestyle choices alongside HRT, and I can honestly put my hand on my heart and say I feel the best I have felt in years. I feel confident, I feel excited, I feel visible and I feel like me for the first time in a long time.

WHY THIS BOOK IS DIFFERENT

In the last few years, there has been a surge in conversations around menopause, which is a wonderful thing, and this has helped many women understand why they are experiencing certain changes and symptoms. However, all too often these conversations are focused on HRT being a magic fix.

Whether you choose to take HRT or not, every woman should know that in order to give yourself the best opportunity to thrive, regardless of your hormone status, introducing more movement into your life, implementing a sensible diet and a sustainable exercise routine that encourages you to lift weights are all crucial.

This book has been written with this in mind and from my own learnt and lived experience. Nothing changed for me until I started lifting weights, and I want to empower you so you can experience the same revelation.

If you commit to following this book's Fitter, Calmer, Stronger in 30 Days Plan, you will soon feel and see the difference and hopefully be motivated to continue making weights a non-negotiable part of your new fitness journey. By implementing these changes today, you will feel the benefits for life, but you need to allow yourself the opportunity to succeed by staying focused and committed to the plan for one month.

Lifting weights will help you find energy and confidence you never knew existed and I want to emphasise that you mustn't be afraid of starting to lift weights. Regular exercise and sensible eating are critical for effectively managing the changing symptoms of the menopause, increasing energy levels and boosting confidence, but it is weights that will add a totally different layer to your life.

This first two parts of the book will explain – without over-complicating things – about what might be happening in your menopause and why you may feel less motivated to start exercising. In part 3, you'll then find the 30-Day Plans to help get you started. When I thought about the structure of the book and how best to help women start, I wanted to make sure they felt supported and not alone when it came to workouts. So, I decided that a follow-along on-demand, real-life 30-Day Plan would be valuable. I myself have purchased books with every intention of doing the workouts, but then not managed to commit to them. The reality is there is nothing more motivating than knowing someone is right there with you, guiding you, encouraging you and working out alongside you, and this is what sets this book apart.

When you get to the workout section, you will have access to a unique QR code that will take you to videos on the 30-day on-demand section. You will have a choice of beginner or inter-mediate/advanced levels so everyone can enjoy the sessions regardless of entry point. The meal plans will sit nicely alongside, ensuring you are nourishing your body – these are not intended for weight loss but to show you how you need to eat well alongside exercise.

Don't be tempted to skip straight to the 30-day exercise and meal plans. Read through the whole book before you get started, as it will help you to understand how all the elements of the Own Your Menopause programme work together so you're more likely to stay on track and make permanent positive changes.

PART 1

What's Happening to Me?

Stop trying to fix your body. It was never broken.

Eve Ensler

I was completely unaware of what was happening to me at the beginning of my story and it wasn't until I was in the throes of perimenopause that I began to understand. My story is not unique, and that scared me, so it is a situation I have set about trying to change.

Many of the women I see and work with are unaware that the menopause has crept up on them as the changes they experience seem to happen gradually over time, bringing many symptoms that come and go. They often find a number of 'unusual' symptoms they have difficulty explaining or understanding where they came from.

It wasn't until I fully understood what menopause was (which I will go into in more detail in Chapter 1) that I was able to make fundamental changes to my exercise programme and then have the fortune to share with my clients. With little understanding of how our declining hormones impact us at this time, many women over-exercise and under-eat, which can harm our hormone health and fitness journeys. I have now trained and supported thousands of women who have all experienced the life-changing magic of lifting weights combined with eating well and they are thriving through, and beyond, what for some can be a difficult life transition.

It is important to acknowledge that the menopause isn't to blame for everything and that naturally as we grow older, our body shape undergoes change. However, our lifestyle choices can significantly impact the pace of these changes. Assessing what measures we can take to support our bodies through menopause and ageing well is crucial.

Rather than trying to resist or fix it, embracing the natural ageing process and working in harmony with our bodies to age gracefully is key. Then not only are we setting ourselves up for success, but we can make menopause a truly positive experience.

We will all be starting this transition from a different place and your journey is unique.

I explain to the women I work with that some of the physiological and metabolic changes they will go through during menopause and beyond, while out of their immediate control, and for the majority not always linear, can still be managed well.

At 57, I thought a menopausal muffin top was with me for life. My daughters had tried to help and they told me wearing a swimming costume is OK, but I wanted to wear a bikini!!! Which I did again after a few weeks. Kate has educated me to see it's not all about the bikini and I have a much more balanced outlook and a better understanding of what I need when it comes to nutrition. Working out with Kate and adding weights to my programme has made me feel accountable, confident, happy and fit. The difference in 5 months is amazing. If I can do it, so can anyone.

Fi

This book will help you see that you have the power to take control. It is you that gets to determine how to live this next chapter of your life by implementing some non-negotiable lifestyle changes to thrive and support the inevitable changes in your body.

CHAPTER 1

What is Menopause?

I am assuming that you have chosen to read this book because it has 'menopause' on the cover and you may already be experiencing some of the symptoms. Perhaps you have even done your own research and have an understanding of what it is you are going through? Maybe you are here because you have tried everything with little success and you want more of a hand-held approach?

Well, firstly you are in the right place. However, I do want to go back over the basics in this journey to getting fitter, calmer and stronger.

Menopause is when the ovaries no longer respond to the hormonal messages sent from the pituitary gland in the brain. This slowly leads to the end of ovulation and the menstrual cycle. As we go through menopause, some women will experience a rollercoaster of emotions as their body tries to adapt to the rise and fall of the hormones involved.

Menopause can also occur when a woman's ovaries are affected by certain treatments, such as chemotherapy or radiotherapy, or when ovaries need to be surgically removed, often during a hysterectomy.

The menopausal transition will affect each woman uniquely. It typically begins between the ages of 45–55, although it can occur earlier. It usually lasts about 7 years but can be as long as 14.

Menopause terminology

Premenopause This starts when a woman begins her reproductive years and ends when she experiences the first symptoms of perimenopause. The beginning of premenopause ties into one's first menstrual cycle.

Perimenopause Women are often unaware that they may be heading towards the menopause. The first stage of this transition is called perimenopause. This can occur between the ages of 45–55 and the average age is 51.

A small number of women – 1 in 100 – will experience the menopause before the age of 40, and an even smaller number – 1 in 1,000 – may go through menopause under 30. There are approximately 13 million women in the UK going through menopause.

In perimenopause, the hormones oestrogen and progesterone begin to fluctuate and decline. The continuous imbalance of these hormones brings about numerous symptoms, causing confusion for many women.

Tracking your symptoms and cycle as soon as you think you could be at this stage is a great way to help you understand why you might be feeling 'out of sorts', but also so you can deliver a more precise picture to your GP should you decide to talk to them about getting help.

Menopause Menopause represents the end stage of a natural transition in a woman's reproductive life. **It is only one day**. This is the day after you haven't had a period for a year, and your periods are officially over.

Postmenopause This refers to the stage after menopause has occurred and you will be in this stage for the
rest of your life. Your hormone levels remain low and if
your periods have stopped for over a year you are now in
postmenopause or postmenopausal. Some of your symptoms may begin to improve because you are no longer
experiencing the rise and fall of the hormones associated
with menopause, but this is not always the case, and
everyone will experience something different. The most
noted symptom improvement is hot flushes, but it is important to remember that no two people are the same.

Medical Menopause If you have to have a
hysterectomy, chemotherapy for certain types of cancer
or medical or surgical treatment for endometriosis, it may
bring about early menopause. The menopause will
happen much faster than it would normally occur, and
your symptoms may be more severe. The effects can be
permanent, depending on the type of treatment and
extent of damage to the ovaries.

Surgical Menopause Surgical menopause is when a
woman goes into menopause as a result of surgery. This
menopause will come on abruptly if you have both
ovaries removed. Surgical menopause is immediate and
permanent.

There are a plethora of hormones that come into play during your
menopause and these have a significant role when it comes to
your physical and psychological changes. It is imperative to
understand the role of hormones in why we experience many
symptoms.

Many of us know the science behind our menstrual cycle from biology lessons, and some will revisit this when trying to have children. This means that usually we learn about this right at the beginning of our menstruation and ovulation cycles, which means we don't remember, or don't have the right information, when we reach menopause.

The main hormones involved in our menstrual cycle are oestrogen, progesterone and testosterone but other hormones, such as follicle-stimulating hormone (FSH) and luteinising hormone (LH), also play a role.

Oestrogen

This is the primary female sex hormone, which plays an essential role in both reproductive and non-reproductive health and is the hormone most responsible for the myriad menopausal symptoms we may experience.

Oestrogen is part of your hormonal (endocrine) system and is mainly produced by the ovaries. It is needed for puberty and breast development, the menstrual cycle, fertility and pregnancy, bone strength and normal cholesterol levels. It also affects other body parts, such as your brain and heart. The luteinizing hormone (LH) and follicle-stimulating hormone (FSH) are produced by the pituitary gland; they promote ovulation and stimulate the ovaries to produce oestrogen and progesterone. These two hormones stimulate the uterus to prepare for possible fertilisation.[1]

As women age, their ovarian response reduces, causing fluctuations in oestrogen and progesterone levels during the perimenopause phase until a woman reaches menopause. During normal menstruation cycles, the levels of oestrogen and progesterone are in balance with each other. However, these levels begin to fall as women approach their mid-thirties to early forties. As we head into menopause and oestrogen deficiency occurs, LH levels increase. Later the FSH is raised and remains high for the rest of life. These raised FSH and low estrogen levels cause the characteristic hot flushes and other symptoms of menopause.[2]

As a result, women may notice a change in their periods. They may be more or less frequent, last longer or be shorter, and may be heavier or lighter. It's not unusual during perimenopause to have missed periods.

The sharp decline in oestrogen, known for causing many of the symptoms associated with menopause, occurs towards the end of the perimenopause. These symptoms can hinder fitness goals and for those who are wanting to start, they may be a barrier to getting going.

It is important to note that, as we will see, implementing an achievable routine including weights alongside a protein-rich diet can help alleviate and manage many of these symptoms.

Progesterone

This is a female steroid hormone derived from cholesterol and primarily made and secreted from the ovaries. Its primary role is to prepare a woman's body for pregnancy and is essential for maintaining the uterine lining.

It plays a vital role in menopause if you take hormone replacement therapy (HRT) (see Chapter 3) because oestrogen alone can cause abnormal uterine lining thickening, which may increase your chances of developing uterine, cervical or vaginal cancer. Progesterone thins the lining of the womb and reduces that risk. If a women has no womb she has no need for extra progesterone.

During the normal menstrual cycle, progesterone works

oppositely to oestrogen to keep both hormones balanced. Oestrogen rises in the first phase of the menstrual cycle to promote the development of an egg, while in the next phase, progesterone takes over, preparing the body for pregnancy or until the period occurs.

However, during perimenopause, levels of oestrogen and progesterone fluctuate. A woman's menstrual cycle is less predictable and low progesterone levels can cause heavier menstrual bleeds. In addition to changes in a woman's menstrual cycle, declining progesterone levels can cause other symptoms such as vaginal dryness because progesterone helps to thicken the mucus in the cervix.

Menopause symptoms can also be caused by declining levels of progesterone because if they no longer balance oestrogen levels, this will cause oestrogen to become dominant before it, too, declines.

Testosterone

This is not just a male hormone, it can also affect your sex drive. Testosterone is produced in the ovaries and the adrenal gland and contributes to our sexual desires and assists and maintains normal metabolic function, muscle and bone strength, mood and cognitive function. Declining testosterone levels can contribute to low libido, changes in cognitive function and mood and may increase the risk of developing osteoporosis.

Unlike progesterone or oestrogen levels, which drop dramatically at the time of menopause, testosterone levels decline slowly as women age.[3]

Testosterone may be prescribed alongside HRT to women who have reduced libido. However, when writing this, testosterone is only readily available on a private prescription. Some women find that it can also help them with stamina and energy, which, when it comes to exercise, can be helpful.

If approached correctly, such as with my 30-Day Plan, weight training during menopause may naturally increase testosterone levels temporarily post-workout.

CHAPTER 2

Menopausal Symptoms

Every woman will go through menopause, but many of us don't realise we are there until we are in the throes of it. Some of you may have been lucky enough to understand this and be ready, but it is understood that almost half of women haven't spoken to their GP surgery about their symptoms. Too often, menopause symptoms are dismissed by GP's, and HRT is not considered and we feel dismissed. When a large number of women face three or more severe symptoms this just doesn't feel fair.

It's not all hot flashes and weight gain. We now know there are over 40 symptoms associated with menopause. Some symptoms are more common than others, and please remember that menopause is different for every woman. You may experience several symptoms at the same time or individually.

These symptoms can significantly impact our daily life, including relationships, social life, family life and work. If we start thinking about how to look after our bodies sooner, we may be able to avoid some of these pitfalls and potentially minimise their impact on our overall health and well-being.

A report from the Fawcett Society published in May 2022,[4] based on data from the largest-ever survey of menopausal and perimenopausal women in the UK, also revealed a shocking lack of support for menopause by healthcare providers and in the workplace:

77%	of women find at least one menopause symptom 'very difficult'
84%	experience trouble sleeping
73%	experience brain fog
69%	experience difficulties with anxiety and depression due to menopause
54%	say they lost interest in sex during menopause
41%	say they have seen menopause or menopause symptoms treated as a joke by people at work
39%	of women who had taken time off due to menopause had cited anxiety or depression as the main reason for their sick note rather than sharing their menopause status

Hot flushes and sweats

A hot flush is the most commonly known menopausal symptom, which has led to much confusion in women who don't experience them and it's important to note that every woman's experience will be different. For those of you experiencing this symptom, you will know it presents as a sudden feeling of warmth in the upper body, usually most intense over the face, neck and chest. Your skin might redden as if you're blushing. It can also cause sweating. If you lose too much body heat, you might feel chilled afterwards.

The frequency and intensity of hot flushes vary – an episode may last between 1–5 minutes. Some women only experience night sweats, a night-time version of hot flushes, which may wake them from sleep. This was one of my worst symptoms and had me changing my pyjamas and bedsheets in the middle of the night.

How often hot flushes occur varies among women, but most women experience them daily.

The good news here is that a regular, moderately intensive workout may help reduce hot flushes by improving the control and stability of your thermoregulatory system.[5]

Anxiety

Experiencing anxiety is relatively common during menopause and is accompanied by a feeling of breathlessness for many women. It can be a terrifying experience that can leave many confused as it tends to creep up slowly out of nowhere.

Anxiety and depression can occur due to falling oestrogen levels, which can change how your brain functions. Studies have shown that oestrogen is linked to brain serotonin levels (the 'happy hormone'). Some women seem to be more susceptible to hormone level changes than others.[6]

If you've suffered from postnatal depression or premenstrual syndrome in the past, the PMT can worsen in perimenopause and you may be more likely to suffer from mood changes during this transition. If you lead a busy life, which many of us do at this time, and you are caring for sick or elderly parents and children on top of your usual to-do list, you may put this symptom down to a general feeling of overwhelm and not put two and two together. One survey showed that 50 per cent of the women interviewed (aged 45–65 and transitioning through menopause) experienced mood changes.[7]

Movement is so beneficial in managing anxiety and increasing energy, which can be low in times of anxiety. Moving your body reduces stress and increases your well-being, confidence and body image.

Irregular periods

The decline in hormones means that ovulation may become more unpredictable. The length of time between periods can be longer or shorter, your flow may be lighter or heavier and some women miss a period altogether.

If you have a persistent change of 7 days or more in the length of your menstrual cycle, you may be in early perimenopause. If you have a space of 60 days or more between periods, you're likely in late perimenopause.

It is important to try and track your cycle because the irregularity may impact your desire to move. Knowing why you feel less energised can help you stay committed to your fitness routine rather than just feeling like it's too much (see Chapter 4).

The likelihood of an irregular cycle and potentially having to manage everything from longer cycles to shorter cycles, spotting and heavy bleeding can be unsettling and frustrating during perimenopause. Periods may also not settle into any obvious patterns, especially as you get closer to menopause.

NOTE
Please see your doctor if bleeding is extremely heavy – you're changing tampons or pads every hour or 2 for 2 or more hours.

Joint and muscle aches

You have oestrogen receptors all over the body, including joints, and declining hormone levels may add to pain caused by inflammation, general wear and tear and just simply ageing. Making lifestyle changes to your diet and exercise routine can help manage these aches and pains and may help to prevent osteopenia, which can lead to osteoporosis.

Fibromyalgia

I often see many women navigating menopause who have had a diagnosis of fibromyalgia. This long-term condition causes pain all over the body. It can also cause extreme tiredness, difficulty sleeping, brain fog, headaches and irritable bowel syndrome, all symptoms that might be confused with menopause, which often means women are dismissed with the wrong diagnosis.

Fibromyalgia can also lead women to stopping movement, but implementing lifestyle changes and incorporating a good exercise plan, including lifting weights, will help alleviate pain.

My top tips if you are experiencing any pain

- Have a magnesium salt bath in the evenings and to incorporate a stretching routine before bed.
- In the morning, allow yourself time to wake up, and then try to repeat the evening stretch.
- If you wanted to look at any supplementation to help, I would recommend vitamin D and magnesium.
- If you are not taking HRT, you might want to consider it if you feel joint and muscle aches hinder you from starting an exercise regime.
- For women who can't or don't want to take HRT, it will be even more important to try to eat a healthy, balanced diet high in fibre with lots of fruit, vegetables and whole grains.

- You should also try to continue with an exercise routine incorporating weight-bearing exercises to strengthen your musculoskeletal system, which will help alleviate joint aches and pains, protect your bones and potentially prevent the onset of osteoporosis. Please remember that quality of movement versus quantity is more important.

The most important thing to remember is that exercise can help you overcome aches and pains and you can build strength regardless of your starting point; you just need to go about exercise differently (see Chapter 5).

Weight gain

Some women experience unexplained weight gain as they go through menopause. As your hormones drop, so does your metabolic rate, which means it is easier to gain weight. Lower testosterone levels during perimenopause and menopause also contribute to slowing down your metabolism, making it harder to shift fat.

Some women try to combat this with increased movement and restriction in calories, which can increase stress on the body and have a negative effect.

If you aren't already moving, this is the time to start. An increase in weight around your middle can leave you more susceptible to diseases like Type 2 diabetes and heart disease.

We tend to store fat around our middle during the menopause because our body recognises declining ovarian oestrogen levels and looks elsewhere for the hormone in a weak form of oestrogen produced by fat cells. The body then tries to create more of this oestrogen by building up fat stores.

Mood fluctuations

Mood swings and fluctuations in menopause can be challenging, and some women find them upsetting. Not everyone will experience the same symptoms, but this is a very common symptom during the perimenopause and menopause.

You may experience a spectrum of emotions – low mood, anxiety, irritability and anger – and feel tearful completely out of the blue. You may also feel totally calm one minute and see red the next, acting completely irrationally. This can be upsetting for you and those around you, who may bear the brunt of your mood swings.

Fatigue

Menopause usually coincides with midlife, which, as mentioned previously, can come with challenges that leave us feeling unusually tired. I see many women who think exercise will tire them even more. The reality is that movement breeds movement. This isn't to say you need to do lots, but I would encourage you to start looking at introducing more movement, especially strength training and weights, into your life. Once you begin to feel the difference, you will feel more motivated.

I would also suggest that you look at your diet to ensure you are eating enough good, nutritious foods to help nourish your body as it goes through this transition. Menopause is not a time to cut out or restrict. As your body experiences these hormonal changes, you must support your hormone health to avoid energy slumps, fatigue and exhaustion.

If you have changed your diet and implemented a sustainable way of moving but you still feel tired, it would be sensible to explain this to your GP.

Body odour

It's not uncommon for women to experience body odour during menopause. A drop in oestrogen levels as you go through menopause can lead to some women having slightly raised testosterone. This can cause you to have more bacteria in your sweat, which may smell more. It is also why many women experience skin changes and acne during menopause.

Your hot flushes can also cause your body to sweat more and often may create a permanent change due to your hormone levels. Many women find that HRT helps with the night sweats that can cause an increase in body odour. For those that don't want to take HRT or can't, you could look at changing your deodorant and wearing cooler, loose clothing at night and in the day. Fans and cooling sprays can also be helpful.

It's really important to note that while you may think you smell horrible, you probably imagine it's worse than it is.

Sleep

The decline in hormones can see our sleep patterns hugely disrupted. The hormones that play a role in hindering sleep are melatonin, oestrogen and progesterone. Add in some night sweats, and you may find that you are only averaging 4–5 hours a night.

Many women also experience insomnia, a chronic difficulty falling asleep or staying asleep more than three nights a week.

Sleep deprivation can increase anxiousness and irritability, impair focus and memory and increase headaches and inflammation, all of which show up liberally as we go through menopause.

Vaginal dryness and atrophy

Clare Bourne Pelvic Health Physio explains that vaginal dryness can be a problem for many postmenopausal women due to decreased oestrogen, which leads to thinner and drier tissues of the vulva and vagina, as well as reduced elasticity. This can also prevent some women from engaging in exercise due to the pain they experience, as dry vulval tissues can be irritated by certain underwear or activewear.

Vaginal dryness, also known as atrophic vaginitis or vaginal atrophy, is a common complaint in menopause. The vaginal tissue becomes thinner and more easily irritated due to the natural decline of your body's oestrogen levels. There is no reason to be embarrassed if you have vaginal dryness that is causing pain during intercourse or exercise. It is imperative to seek help if this is stopping you from progressing in maintaining your fitness levels or preventing you from starting. Both conditions can be addressed if you seek help from your GP. You may be prescribed a low-dose vaginal oestrogen cream or pessary that works to replace the oestrogen that you are lacking, and this is applied directly into your vagina using an applicator. Most of these are prescribed daily for two weeks and then a couple of times a week thereafter.

Pelvic floor issues

Your pelvic floor muscles help support your pelvic organs (uterus, bladder and bowel). As perimenopause progresses, you may experience increased leaks of urine with coughing, sneezing, laughing or exercising as decreased oestrogen levels contribute to changes of the pelvic floor muscles, alongside the natural loss of skeletal muscle as we age, called sarcopenia.

Weakness of these muscles may also contribute to pelvic organ prolapse, where there is a descent of one or more of the pelvic organs (bladder, uterus or bowel) down into the vagina. This is often the result of changes to the pelvic floor muscles, as well as to the connective tissue and ligaments that support the pelvic organs. Women often experience prolapse as a heaviness or dragging sensation in the vagina day-to-day or during or after exercise.

To prevent this from happening, or to help if you do have prolapse symptoms, you should look at focusing on working these muscles as part of your routine, alongside preventing or treating any constipation you might be experiencing. Straining to do a poo can cause or worsen a prolapse and prolapse symptoms.

To strengthen your pelvic floor muscles, try this:

1. Sit comfortably and think about holding in wind or squeezing your anus.
2. Bring this squeeze forwards towards your pubic bone. Then fully release it.
3. Try and do this 10 times in a row, fully releasing between each squeeze.
4. Now try to hold the contraction. Contract the muscles in the same way (squeezing around your anus and bringing this forwards to your pubic bone) and hold this squeeze for up to 10 seconds while you breathe in and out. If 10 seconds feels too long to start with, then reduce this to 3–4 seconds and build up from there. Repeat this 10 times as well.
5. If you are experiencing symptoms of incontinence or prolapse, try and do 10 of each type of squeeze three times a day.
6. Start doing these lying or sitting, but once you are confident, try and do them standing.

When it comes to lifting weights and exercising, you must have good instruction and lift weights properly. A simple principle that can be helpful when thinking about our pelvic floor through movement is to exhale on the effort of the moment. As we breathe out, there is a natural activation of the pelvic floor muscles. Maintaining a healthy weight is also important for the pelvic floor, as being overweight can worsen pelvic floor symptoms by increasing the pressure on the muscles and organs.

Menopausal symptoms checker

Below is a table of the most common menopausal symptoms you might experience. Please start tracking them so you can have a good picture to show your GP should you decide to approach them for HRT. It is also important to track so you can see how exercise and diet play a role and what might alleviate or trigger symptoms. The more knowledge you have of your own menopause, the better equipped you will be to manage it.

SYMPTOM	YES	NO	DETAILS	FREQUENCY
HEADACHES				
ANXIETY				
LOW MOOD				
WEIGHT GAIN				
HEART PALPITATIONS				
ANGER				
TEARFULNESS				
BRAIN FOG				
CYCLE CHANGES				
LOSS OF LIBIDO				
POOR CONCENTRATION				
NO MOTIVATION				
LACK OF CONFIDENCE				
FEELING ALONE				
DEPRESSION				

NIGHT SWEATS				
HOT FLUSHES				
BURNING MOUTH				
DRY ITCHY SKIN				
SLEEPLESSNESS				
FEELING DIZZY				
TINNITUS				
RESTLESS LEGS				
BLOATING				
JOINT PAIN				
MUSCLE PAIN				
FATIGUE				
VAGINAL SYMPTOMS				
URINARY SYMPTOMS				
ALLERGIES				
BLOCKED SINUS				

CHAPTER 3

HRT

Hormone replacement therapy, or HRT, is a treatment to relieve symptoms of the menopause. It replaces hormones that are at a lower level as you go through menopause.

For some women, HRT can help manage severe symptoms, BUT it is not a stand-alone measure and you must consider your lifestyle choices alongside taking it if this is your informed decision. My 30-Day Plan is designed with this in mind.

HRT was introduced in the 1960s but didn't gain real popularity until the 1990s. It has had its ups and downs, which has sadly caused much frustration and confusion for women. The Women's Health Initiative (WHI) produced some data in 2005 that caused unnecessary concern amongst many healthcare professionals and had a major impact on women, creating a fear of HRT that is still evident today. Despite numerous studies since highlighting that for most women the benefits do outweigh the risks, there are many who are still unsure about making this choice.

In fact, even after my own diagnosis, and despite the fact it had taken almost 6 months to get one, I was still unsure about taking HRT. I think deep down I kept thinking my symptoms would disappear and this wasn't menopause – apparently this is another common symptom!

I decided to just try it because if it didn't work or I didn't want to carry on, I knew I could just stop. With my night sweats, rage and anxiety at an all-time high, I took the plunge.

If I am honest, my symptoms didn't disappear overnight and it was very much a case of finding the right balance. You do need a good doctor who understands HRT for this. And please remember that everyone's experience of menopause is unique and that HRT is very much your own journey too.

After my 3-month review we did a little tweaking, but with my symptoms still having a negative impact, I started to do my own research on what I could do to support my body better through making lifestyle changes. What happened next was amazing and this is why I am so passionate about this book.

HRT is not a silver bullet – you need to implement non-negotiable lifestyle changes too.

Types of HRT

Oestrogen replacement

Dr Naomi Potter from Menopause Care Clinic has kindly provided us with evidence-based information on Hormone Replacement Therapy (HRT) and why for some women it can be beneficial.[8] This is considered safest when taken through the skin (rather than via the mouth) because it avoids being metabolised in the liver. This is known as the transdermal route instead of the oral route.

Oestrogen is typically available in a patch, spray or gel form, which all deliver the same hormone when prescribed. It's up to the patient's preference based on guidance from their doctor and the product's availability.

The gel can be found in a pump dispenser or disposable sachet. You should apply daily to the skin of the leg, arm, buttock or tummy and allow it to dry for absorption.

The patch is a small, sticky transparent 'plaster' applied to the skin and changed every 3 days. Different patch options are available, with most containing only oestrogen (some contain oestrogen and progesterone).

The spray is applied directly to your skin, where the dose corresponds to the number of sprays you have been prescribed.

Progesterone

This is important to use in women with a uterus (i.e. those without a hysterectomy) in conjunction with oestrogen HRT.

If oestrogen alone is used, the womb's lining (endometrium) can thicken, which after prolonged exposure can lead to cellular changes and the risk of those developing into cancer. Progesterone helps prevent this.

Progesterone can be delivered in a number of ways, but preferred routes are either Utrogestan, the Mirena coil or combined patch.

While the coil can be convenient as it stays in place for 5 years, some women prefer not to use it.

Utrogestan needs to be taken regularly and is considered the most advantageous way of getting progesterone as it is a body identical hormone. Women typically experience fewer side effects. If you choose Utrogestan, there are two methods of taking it: continuous and cyclical. Women in the perimenopause usually take it cyclically, for approximately 2 weeks of their cycle, and this involves having a bleed. Postmenopausal women take it every day in a continuous (bleed-free) regime. Taking progesterone at night can aid sleep.

The small increased risk of breast cancer in women who take HRT is related to the type of progestogen in the HRT (progestogens are a class of synthetic forms of progesterone). Taking Utrogestan does not appear to be associated with an increased risk of breast cancer for the first five years. After this time, the risk of breast cancer is very low. Even for women taking the older types of progestogens, the risk of breast cancer is very low. The level of increased risk with the older types of progestogens is similar to the level of risk of breast cancer in women who are overweight or who drink around two glasses of wine daily.

Testosterone

This is also a female hormone and the decline can impact on your symptoms. GP guidance is usually to wait to see if menopausal symptoms resolve following oestrogen replacement first. If following a blood test your symptoms remain and testosterone levels are low, your doctor may discuss the use of testosterone.

Used at physiologically female doses, it should not cause any masculine side effects. The only product currently available in the UK designed for female use is AndroFeme, but only on private prescription. Male products are not currently licenced for menopause but are available off licence.

If you choose HRT, it is available on the NHS via your GP and in private clinics. When you start HRT, your symptoms can take a few days to a few months to improve. You can experience side effects in the first few months, but these mostly settle with time.

Breast cancer

Managing menopause in women with a history of breast cancer is always more challenging. You may have been on treatment to block oestrogen and therefore HRT may not be an option.

Menopause specialist Dr Naomi Potter has outlined some non-hormonal medication:

- **Oxybutynin** This can be helpful with hot flushes. Side effects can be a dry mouth and nausea.
- **Clonidine** This can help with hot flushes, especially in women taking Tamoxifen. However, it can cause side effects such as nausea, headaches and dizziness and must be used cautiously in women who already take blood pressure medication.
- **Venlafaxine** In terms of hot flushes, Venlafaxine has the most convincing evidence of a positive outcome and can also help with mood.
- **Paroxetine and Fluoxetine** These can be useful for hot flushes and mood disturbance, but neither should be used with Tamoxifen as they can reduce its efficacy.
- **Gabapentin** Can be helpful with hot flushes and mood disturbance. It can cause nausea and gastric upset.

While HRT can and has helped many women, I want all women to have the means to alleviate their menopausal symptoms within their immediate reach. Every woman can build their own personal toolkit to manage their menopause holistically. This means taking a whole approach to thriving, not simply relying on HRT. HRT does NOT work on its own and, in fact, for some women it doesn't work at all.

CHAPTER 4

Menstruation and Its Impact on Exercise

Understanding your menstrual cycle when you exercise during your perimenopause is important because it can impact your body from head to toe, which in turn may impact your sessions.

Many women assume that to be diagnosed as perimenopausal they should no longer have periods. This is not the case. If you are experiencing many of the symptoms of menopause but have periods, you can still be considered perimenopausal.

I encourage all women in perimenopause to track their cycles as best they can. It's also worth mentioning that if you have the coil, you will still experience hormonal fluctuations because oestrogen is the primary hormone responsible for these fluctuations.

Listening to your body and noting your physiological symptoms will be instrumental in changing the narrative towards yourself when it comes to exercise. If you feel like you're not entirely up to the task you've set, it's important to be kind to yourself and remember the changes you are going through. Your hormones may be playing a role in how you're feeling and the simple fact is that when your hormones are doing their own thing, you cannot do anything about it other than learn to work alongside them. It's possible that you haven't realised how much your hormones affect your fitness routine. Some days you may feel energised and ready to tackle a marathon; on others, getting out of bed seems like a challenge.

Some of you may find that your cycles are as regular as clock-work; others will begin to see changes and find it hard to pinpoint where they are in the cycle. For me, the irregularity was an indication something was changing. Physical and mental transitions can be challenging, but knowing the reasons behind our feelings and comfortably moving our bodies can make obstacles more manageable. We can also improve our mood and increase our energy levels.

The menstrual cycle

Phase 1

This is the first day of your period. In this first or reset phase, your LH (luteinising hormone), oestrogen, progesterone and testosterone, the primary hormones that control your menstrual cycle, are all at their lowest point.

For many women having their period is not the most comfortable time of the month, and it can bring about numerous symptoms. However, as menstruation gets underway, PMS symptoms subside, your body temperature returns to a more normal level, and some of your energy begins to creep back.

Impact on exercise: LOW ENERGY
You have your period, therefore, you will likely feel slightly lacking in energy. You turn up to your regular class, but don't feel like it or haven't done as well as you hoped. This is okay, and the reason will be because of your hormones. You are still making progress, but today just isn't your day – and that is OK.

As you head towards the end of this phase and into the follicular phase, you will feel more capable and able to add more intensity.

What to do: Gentle yoga, walking, stretching or Pilates may be best right now. If you have the energy for higher-intensity exercise, go for it.

Phase 2: the follicular phase

The follicular phase, including the ovulation period, is a great time to start thinking about your progress and strength training. During the follicular phase, the body produces more oestrogen. You might feel like you have a higher tolerance for pain or increasing endurance levels due to this steady rise. Your body is also more likely to use muscle glycogen to fuel exercise. Renourish and refuel with good high-carb meals before and after your workout to optimise your training and aid recovery.

Impact on exercise: ENERGY INCREASING
Your oestrogen levels are beginning to rise. You feel your energy increasing and are likely to find exercise more appealing and possible.

What to do: It's an excellent time to focus on your strength training and a great time to build muscle because your physical strength is at its best. You may also feel a little more creative and dynamic, so this is the time to add some weights to your workout.

Phase 3: the ovulation phase

As you ovulate, your strength levels will still be relatively high, and you may even notice this. If you want to set a personal best, now might be the time to try. One study published in the *Journal of Physiology*[9] noted that ovulating women showed an 11 per cent increase in quadriceps and handgrip strength.

However, you are also at a higher risk of injury during this time. Your oestrogen, FSH and LH levels reach their highest peak and your metabolism is beginning to increase, so you might feel a bit more peckish. Understanding and addressing this means that if you do need to add more calories, you can get these from a balanced mix of protein, carbs and fats rather than sugary alternatives, as your insulin sensitivity is declining.

Impact on exercise: PEAK ENERGY

The release of the egg from the ovary mid-cycle may see you experiencing an increase in energy levels and strength. It is the oestrogen, FSH and LH peak that can cause this increase, allowing you to feel able to put more effort into your workouts.

What to do: This is an ideal time to try a HIIT or spin class, maybe even with friends, as you're also more sociable. Take advantage of your increased strength and train hard but pay attention to your body, noting how it feels, as it is also a time when injuries can occur, so be sure to warm up and cool down properly.

Phase 4: the luteal phase

During this phase, your body temperature tends to be higher than normal, and you may find that you are reaching the point of exhaustion or feeling more fatigued a little sooner than in the previous weeks. You may also be retaining excess water, making it a little bit more uncomfortable to work out, and you may feel sluggish.

Your serotonin production is lower in this phase, so you may find yourself craving high-carbohydrate foods and sugary snacks.

Try to be aware of this because your instinct will be to grab those foods, whereas it would be better to go for foods high in protein to offset these cravings.

Impact on exercise: ENERGY DECLINE

After experiencing a boost in energy and successfully meeting your personal goals, it's common to suddenly feel like your efforts are not producing the desired outcome, leading to decreased confidence. If you feel less energetic, consider engaging in low-intensity cardio training paired with moderate strength exercises. When you're feeling exhausted and irritable, try adjusting your routine and incorporating activities like yoga, Pilates, dancing or any other activity that interests you.

Additionally, it's worth noting that your metabolic rate may have increased, leading to a higher likelihood of craving sugary foods and having an increased appetite.

What to do: LISS, yoga, Pilates, jogging, lighter weights.

Summary

- Women will experience hormone imbalance as they enter and transition through to menopause due to declining oestrogen, progesterone and testosterone levels. Many of the 40+ symptoms can be managed with exercise and diet.

- The average age of menopause is 51, but it can take some women up to 14 years to go through perimenopause.

- These hormonal changes will impact a woman's physical and mental health to varying degrees during perimenopause with a range of symptoms experienced, many of which can be managed holistically.

- Menopause often coincides with midlife, which can be a time when we find ourselves juggling family, home and work life and elderly or sick parents. Many of the menopause symptoms can make life that extra bit harder and many women feel lost, invisible and unheard. We may be inclined to put our own health and well-being on the back burner.

- Many women are still unaware that much of what they may be feeling is due to the decline in hormones through menopause. Empowering ourselves with information and implementing healthy lifestyle changes is key.

• Now is the time to start thinking about your own movement. Knowing that the symptoms you are experiencing are due to menopause helps you understand better what it is you need to do to help you get back to feeling better, and how exercise and diet has a fundamental role to play in doing so.

PART 2

Owning Your Movement

Take care of your body. It's the only place you have to live.

Jim Rohn

We have looked at the biology of menopause, the symptoms and how HRT might help with management, but that is only part of Owning Your Menopause. I have first-hand experience of how HRT alone might not work. And even if it does for you, without making lifestyle changes I can almost guarantee it will only work initially. What was transformative for me were the other changes I made when it came to movement and diet.

I have seen so many women who have always been really fit and healthy suddenly struggle to keep up their usual routines. In fact, I was one of them. With the belief that HIIT training was my only option, my body began to feel tired and I was experiencing more aches and pains. This is a common complaint from midlife women and the reason we must look at changing the way we move.

If this sounds like you, in fact even if it doesn't, strength training with weights is the only answer for not only managing many of your menopausal symptoms, but also helping with weight loss or maintenance. This is why it is so important and is the basis of the 30-Day Plan.

Whatever your starting point, you can come on this journey. Some of you will already have an understanding or have a routine in place that may or may not be working. Others of you will be starting at the beginning. Wherever you are, empowering yourself with the knowledge of how important adding more movement – walking, running, Pilates, gardening – is at this time will equip you for any challenges you may face. For those of you who are new to exercise and for whom the idea of lifting weights fills you with fear, under my guidance and following the plan you will find a love for this type of movement as you begin to feel the positive changes associated with strength training as an integral part of your exercise routine.

I work with so many women who have always seen exercise as a means to an end and that end is usually a weight-related goal, implying that movement is only worthwhile if it helps them slim down or burn calories. This has significantly impacted their mental and future physical health because they overlook the actual benefits of exercise and, for many, it makes exercise a chore and not a pleasure. I would love for every woman to have the opportunity to learn to love to exercise for all the benefits it will provide them as they age well and build strong minds and bodies.

We know that a woman's bone density reaches its peak at the age of 30, and their muscle mass declines from 35, so the sooner we start adding weights to our routine the better.[10] By lifting weights, you may also prevent the early onset of osteoporosis, which is associated with the decline in oestrogen, so see this as your opportunity to try things differently, a time of transition that will help you prepare for the next stage of your life.

CHAPTER 5

Reframing Your Mindset

I think one of the greatest tragedies in our lives – in women's lives – is the time, the effort, the energy, the passion that we've wasted on not being able to accept our own bodies.

Emma Thompson

Menopause can be a wonderful opportunity to grow, learn and understand the role of moving the body because it feels good and helps you build a stronger, more resilient body. It is the perfect time to reframe and evaluate many of your preconceived notions about exercise and diet.

I think one of the most significant underlying issues for many of us is that growing up, we weren't fed images of strong women like we see today, which has led to many of us battling with our self-confidence. In the past, magazines often implied that being thin or skinny was the desirable representation of a strong and successful woman. This meant that movement was never really a pleasure, instead, it was tied up with a mixture of feelings. It was always a means to an end, more often than not a weight-loss goal, maybe even a punishment.

It can be hard to unravel years of negative self-talk and relearn disciplines that have controlled our behaviour and mindset around movement and food. Maybe some of you developed a dislike for sports growing up. Getting picked last for teams or finishing last in a race on sports day is, for many of us, a nightmare in childhood and can affect how you perceive your physical capability and exercise itself.

Imagine having grown up with the option to have moved because it just felt good and it was enjoyable, with no pressure to achieve anything specific. It would have been life-changing for many, and this is something I would like you to learn.

If this resonates with you, take time to reframe this mindset and train your mind to understand the new set of rules you are putting into place to future-proof your body and optimise your well-being.

Learn to move because it feels good, and you're grateful you can. If you aren't already, you must start doing the movement you enjoy and stop doing the things you don't.

Intuitive Movement is about taking an approach to exercise that encourages you to tune into your body and listen to what it needs. It can help you to unlearn the idea that exercise merely exists as a means to shrink your body and instead allows you to reframe your mindset to see that movement is there to nourish your mind and body for longevity and strength. You are choosing an activity that YOU enjoy and feels good and not choosing exercise for how many calories it burns.

I'd love you to try this and see how it makes you feel:

Close your eyes and think about how you like to move your body. What makes you feel happy? What feels possible? What would you like to do that would have an impact on your mood and overall well-being? Think about pleasurable ways to move for enjoyment and remove any 'weight' related thoughts.

Movement should bring you joy and fulfilment. Mantras such as 'no pain, no gain', 'pain is temporary' and even phrases like 'the only workout you regret is the one you did not do' place an unnecessary emphasis on working out because you have to rather than because you want to and it feels good.

How we grow old and what this looks like is down to us. We get to determine (to a large extent) what the next chapter of our life looks like, which is why moving while listening to our bodies is imperative. While we can't prevent any pre-determined disease, we can give ourselves the best chance of dealing with any diagnosis we might receive.

Start listening to your body and focus on movement for your bone, heart, muscle and brain health (see Chapter 6) and try to put any aesthetic goals aside.

CHAPTER 6

The Health Benefits of Moving in Menopause

I see menopause as the start of the next fabulous phase of a woman's life. Now is a time to tune in to our bodies and embrace this new chapter.

Kim Cattrall

Menopause should not be seen as it is by many as a signal of impending decline, but as a wonderful new beginning where you take control of your health by implementing positive lifestyle changes. We must do all we can at this life stage to prevent the onset of age and menopause-related diseases.

As a PT, I was already aware of the benefits of exercise but once I started digging into the research a bit more, I realised that not only was movement a non-negotiable part of the menopause journey, but what we do and how we move is just as important. My own experience is a testament to this as are the women I work with.

I have seen first-hand from working with women who have never exercised the transformative power of incorporating exercise into their lives and making it a daily habit, a non-negotiable:

Your workouts helped me mentally and physically through the tough, traumatic break-up of a relationship and through being furloughed and lost in my life. Being 42 and a single mum again totally lost me and I was in a very dark place. I can't thank you enough. You have been part of my journey, helping me find strength within myself and learning to use and love weights. Getting fitter and stronger and believing in myself a little more. Still working on this. Thank you,

Jenny

I have also had clients who have struggled with crippling joint pain, anxious that movement will exacerbate the pain and other symptoms they are experiencing:

I LOVE the Owning Your Menopause (OYM) platform. After suffering hideous aches and pains in my joints and muscles, I did start HRT but it wasn't enough, so I signed up to OYM and within a month those symptoms (and many others) completely vanished. I was astonished! I'm 51 and I felt the difference in my strength and mobility after 15 days. Fast-forward 3 months and I'm running better than ever now thanks to the combo of HRT and OYM strength training. I'm also enjoying dressing up in all my fancy gear again – fitness and frocks.

Here's to us all running and dancing into our 80s, 90s and beyond!

Annie

An effective workout is not determined by the amount of sweat produced, your inability to move the next day, or the amount of time it's taken. Any movement is beneficial, but it does need to elevate the heart rate at least 3–4 times a week. Ideally, you will also add some resistance to those sessions because this can help you use your time efficiently and will ensure you get the best results.

Exercise is essential to live a healthy and fulfilling life into old age and it is medically proven that people who do regular physical activity, especially as they age, have a lower risk of:
- coronary heart disease and stroke
- Type 2 diabetes
- bowel cancer
- breast cancer in women
- early death
- osteoarthritis
- hip fracture
- falls (among older adults)
- depression
- dementia

Having discussed the significance of staying active during meno-pause, let's look at how movement can help our physical and mental health.

Bone health

During the menopause, oestrogen levels decline, which can lead to increased bone loss because oestrogen helps slow down the natural breakdown of bone. Twenty per cent of bone loss can occur during menopause, and around 1 in 10 women over 60 are affected by osteoporosis, a health condition that weakens bones and makes them more likely to break.[11] Note that your bone mass peaks at 30, and if it's already below ideal levels, any bone loss during menopause may result in osteoporosis. Adding strength training, like we will do in the 30-Day Plan, will allow your body to build stronger bones. This is done by placing them under considerably more resistance than normal day-to-day activities, promoting better bone growth and strength.

Some women may be fortunate enough to have the opportunity to have a DEXA scan.[12] This bone density scan uses low-dose X-rays to see how dense (or strong) your bones are and to diagnose or assess your risk of osteoporosis, As well as being quick and painless, a bone density scan is more effective than regular X-rays in identifying low bone density.

If you cannot get a DEXA scan, please see your GP and say you would like a FRAX® score, which should be available to anyone who has a concern or would just like to have peace of mind. If you have had fracture or a broken bone that is unexplained, you should push your GP for this. FRAX®[13] is a sophisticated risk assessment instrument developed by the University of Sheffield that helps to identify people who may be at risk of developing osteoporosis. Personal details (such as weight, medication history, smoking history and family history) are entered to predict whether someone is at risk of developing osteoporosis in the next 10 years. This information can help your doctor decide whether further action needs to be taken.

Your bone health can be protected with proper nutrition, including adequate calcium and vitamin D.

One in three women over 50 years will sustain a hip fracture, which can have severe consequences for their health.

For good bone health and osteoporosis prevention, exercise is fundamental, especially adding resistance and weight training.

Joint health

As oestrogen declines, it can affect the joints and connective tissues, which may cause pain for many women.

If you already suffer from joint pain, high-impact activities that aggravate this pain should be avoided, at least in the short term. You can still do plenty of exercises to build strength in your joints. If you want to be able to do high-impact exercise, the key is to introduce it slowly and listen to your symptoms to find the right intensity for you.

Exercise increases strength, makes moving easier, and it reduces joint pain and helps fight tiredness. We should all move, but this is even more important for people with joint aches and pains, even those with arthritis. There's no need to run a marathon or swim for miles. Even moderate exercise can ease pain and help you stay at a healthy weight.

Movement will help to prevent and relieve pain in your joints – motion is lotion.

You will feel less stiff and fatigued if you continue to move, plus you will release feel-good endorphins, which help you manage pain and see that movement is beneficial in supporting joint health.

Muscle health

As we go through menopause, our muscle mass can decline by 3–5 per cent per year, coupled with hormonal fluctuations, which also hinder muscle gain.[14]

The decline in muscle mass is called sarcopenia. Once we hit the age of 30, our muscles naturally start to shrink. Building muscle will help you stay strong and avoid fragility as you age. It may also help you live longer because muscle mass is inversely associated with the risk of death.

With this in mind, there's never been a better time to focus on improving your muscle mass.

Hormonal fluctuations hinder muscle gain, so it is essential to start looking at exercise's role and how we can protect our future health by building lean muscle.

- Muscle helps manage blood sugar.
- Muscle builds strength and stamina.
- Muscle supports your joints.
- Building muscle builds bone.
- Muscle helps you control body fat.

Heart health

Many people think that heart disease is a man's disease. It isn't, and after the age of 50, nearly half of all deaths in women are due to some form of cardiovascular disease.

When women reach the age of 50, their risk for heart disease can increase dramatically if they aren't keeping the heart strong and healthy. This is done not only through exercise but by having a balanced, nutritious diet.

Oestrogen has a role in protecting against coronary artery disease by controlling cholesterol levels and reducing fatty plaque build-up inside the artery walls. If we don't exercise and move the body at this time, we leave ourselves more vulnerable once oestrogen declines.

NHS guidelines suggest 150 minutes of exercise a week can significantly reduce your chances of developing heart-related issues.[15] In fact, recent research suggests that 4,000 steps could be enough to significantly reduce your risk of death.[16] Researchers found that the health benefits continue to increase as people walked more, and every increase of 500 steps a day was associated with a 7 per cent reduction in cardiovascular disease.

Heart disease is the second biggest cause of death amongst postmenopausal women in the UK.

A healthy lifestyle goes a long way in preventing heart disease in women.

Being active or exercising regularly helps improve how well the heart pumps blood through your body.

Brain health

Dr Lisa Mosconi has carried out some really interesting research on brain health, highlighting that our brains produce oestrogen and the important role it plays in day-to-day brain functions.

Dr Mosconi says, 'Cognitive challenges can be common during the transition into menopause, including symptoms such as forgetfulness and delayed verbal memory, reduced verbal processing speed and impaired verbal learning, all of which can be pretty scary.'[17] This rings true and I have even found myself in the car driving and drawing a complete blank on my destination.

Exercise can help you think, learn, problem-solve, manage emotions and support mental health. It can also reduce your risk of cognitive decline, including dementia. It is believed that cognitive decline is almost twice as common in adults who are inactive compared to those who are active.

Exercise improves your memory and brain function.

It improves blood flow to your brain.

It helps prevent neurological conditions.

It decreases your brain fog.

Mental health

It's common for women to experience mental health problems due to the hormone changes during menopause. Exercise has so many benefits to help manage anxiety and depression as we go through menopause.

Many people still believe that hot flushes and anger are the signs to look out for, but my own experience of menopause was very much one that impacted my mental health, which is not to be overlooked. You may feel more anxious, irritable and sad. If you are forgetting things, this can lead to loss of self-esteem and confidence.

Many women experiencing menopause or perimenopause will have problems with sleeping. Lack of sleep and tiredness can also worsen symptoms, including irritability, inability to concentrate and anxiety.

Exercise releases chemicals like endorphins and serotonin, which will improve your mood, so it is really important to try to get movement in, even if it feels like the last thing on your mind. Movement can also get you outside, reduce loneliness and isolation, and put you in touch with other people, which can have a huge effect on your mood.

If you exercise regularly, it can reduce your stress and the symptoms of mental health conditions like depression, anxiety or schizophrenia. It can also help with recovery from mental health issues.

It can also improve your sleep, which is important in many different ways.

Confidence

Forty per cent of women consider leaving their jobs due to a lack of confidence and many question their ability on the job as they try to navigate their menopause alone. Some women are even unaware the symptoms they are experiencing are down to menopause due to a distinct lack of education and support in the workplace.[18]

Not only do some women have a crisis of confidence in the workplace, but many also feel lost and unseen in close relationships.

Loss of confidence is common during the menopause transition and is connected with several other symptoms of menopause. Anxiety or fatigue can stop you from socialising or seeing friends, and many women withdraw from life and feel more isolated. Some develop a distorted body image, which can lead to feelings of doubt and, again, a loss of confidence, preventing them from participating in daily activities.

Try to see exercise as a way to connect with other women who can support and understand, so that you keep moving and stay connected. Physical activity can also help manage emotions and demonstrate your body's capabilities despite insecurities. It can change your perception of yourself and give you the confidence to enjoy activities you once loved.

Exercise can help you to feel strong, which can enhance your levels of confidence.

Exercise can give you a sense of achievement, which will boost your endorphins and self-worth.

Movement will also make you feel strong, which in turn allows you to feel like you could do more and socialise again.

Increased energy

Have you ever had that moment in the afternoon when you feel like you're completely exhausted? It used to happen to me all the time, leaving me wondering how I would make it through the rest of the day.

Increasing physical activity can actually help raise your energy levels and it also boosts the oxygen circulation inside your body.

Movement can increase energy levels and help with the afternoon lull, especially if you eat the right foods to help you get through the energy dips.

If you feel the afternoon dip, my advice is to get outside if you can and go for a little walk to help boost your energy.

Better sleep

Sleep deprivation can play havoc with your hormones and significantly impact your mood (see Chapter 14). We already know that the decline in hormones can disrupt our sleep patterns but add in some sweats and you may find that you are only averaging 4–5 hours a night, well below the recommendations.

Exercising improves sleep for many people.[19] Specifically, moderate to vigorous exercise can increase sleep quality for adults by reducing sleep onset – or the time it takes to fall asleep – and decreasing the time they lie awake at night. Additionally, physical activity can help alleviate daytime sleepiness and, for some people, reduce the need for sleep medications.

While specific research varies, health professionals agree that a good night's sleep can help you feel well-rested and more motivated to exercise the following day.

People who exercise claim to sleep better than people who do not.

A 10-minute walk each day can improve your sleep quality.

Sleep plays a significant role in almost every system of the body.

Preventing injury

A real cause for concern is sustaining an injury as we age, which can prevent us from carrying out our day-to-day activities. If we have a good base level of fitness and strength and our body is mobile, we may be able to maintain balance if we fall. Or if we do fall, our bones might be strong enough to avoid breaking. Not only that, but if we were to get an injury and didn't have a good base level, it can take us longer to recover.

Exercise can help prevent injury by offering protective, preventative benefits and future-proofing your body.

Reducing cancers

Many women I see have concerns about diseases beyond their immediate control as they age, and for many of us cancer presents a real fear. Drawing on my own experiences, I know this has been a huge factor in driving me to take better care of myself and make some positive changes to decrease any risks.

Keeping a healthy weight lowers your risk of 13 different cancer types. This includes two of the most common types of cancer (breast and bowel) and three of the hardest-to-treat cancers (pancreatic, oesophageal and gallbladder).[20]

Being physically active lowers bowel and breast cancer risk by helping us maintain a healthy weight. There's also evidence that exercising can directly prevent these cancers in ways unrelated to our weight.

Being very active can boost your immune system, making it work more effectively and allowing the body to get better at spotting cells that could become cancerous. It can then remove these cells before they cause harm.

CHAPTER 7

How to Start and Make It Stick

Sometimes the bravest and most important thing you can do is just show up.

Brené Brown

One of the most common things I see as a PT is women quitting an exercise programme or an unwillingness to start as they go through menopause. They are overwhelmed not only with life but with the confusing amount of misinformation.

Many women become self-conscious and insecure, leading to a lack of motivation to pursue what they used to enjoy. Other women are unsure how to begin and develop a fear that will hinder them from starting. Some begin comparing themselves to those around them, which means they become even more self-conscious and fearful to start.

Some of the symptoms of menopause can be debilitating and I have seen many women, myself included, try to manage crippling joint pain and muscle fatigue. No woman should have to live with this pain and it can be a huge barrier to movement because our instinct tells us to rest, when really 'motion is lotion', and finding the right way to move will have multiple benefits.

I have worked with women who are so exhausted that they need to go back to bed in a matter of hours upon waking, which impacts their physical and mental well-being. If you are in this phase, you could be a candidate for HRT, but as I mentioned earlier, this book will empower you to see what YOU can start changing immediately.

Procrastination, fear of change and a lack of understanding may also prevent you from focusing on your future health. Making excuses and rationalising your behaviour can impede your progress, so when you make an excuse, pause and think about why you're doing this.

Remember that movement will breed movement. As you begin to feel more confident, you will find more ways to keep fit, strong and mobile.

Common obstacles

Lack of time

A barrier to starting or continuing with a fitness programme is that many women are time-poor. I understand how hard this is. We are juggling many balls and making time for ourselves can seem over-whelming. However, carving out time is important because you will feel more able to cope mentally with the challenges you face, and you will also be better at supporting those around you. Setting the alarm 15 minutes before your usual waking time can be enough time to allow some movement and time for yourself. In the 30-Day Plan, I have put in some shorter workouts to enable this, so please give it a go.

Muscle and joint pain

This is a common obstacle that women face and is instrumental in hindering progress for many. If you find this symptom especially crippling and you have already implemented lifestyle changes, you could see your GP and talk about HRT. For some women, this may be needed, but that doesn't mean stopping the positive changes. If you are new to exercise and experiencing aches and pains from menopause, please know that moving your body will be instrumental in lubricating the joints and building muscle, which can go a long way to relieving the pain. Don't let muscle and joint pain stop you from starting or continuing exercise.

No motivation

Many of us may find the symptoms of menopause hit us like a cyclical rollercoaster that can find us lacking in motivation. This is likely to come from placing unrealistic expectations on yourself and when it doesn't go to plan, or you aren't forgiving of yourself, you lose motivation. It's common to start a new regime enthusiastically and have all the best intentions on a Sunday evening, but if you have made your programme unachievable, you will have no motivation or desire to continue.

The 30-Day Plan will help you see what is realistic to change and will set you up for success by creating good habits.

Low energy

We know that one of the symptoms of menopause is low energy, which is often associated with poor sleep and night sweats. It can also indicate too much sugar or a glucose spike. It's no wonder that some women are too tired to move. The good news is that if you start moving even just a little, you will increase your chances of a better night's sleep, which could give you more energy to move.

In Chapter 19 we will look at the importance of managing your sugar intake, which will also help manage your energy.

Too late

With a distinct lack of representation of women going through menopause and midlife on social media or in the press, many believe it is too late to make changes and this can often be a driver for not trying. It is never too late to start, and with heart disease being one of the biggest causes of death among women postmenopausally, I would encourage you to start today.

The most important thing to remember is that you can start regardless of age or starting point. You can also make as much progress at home as you can in a gym, but you do need to make a small investment in some weights, ideally dumbbells. The 30-Day Plan will guide you through and give you the confidence to carry on. It is very common to feel nervous, but when you do feel like this, please remember everyone started somewhere and you are not alone. So don't let this be a barrier to optimising your well-being.

Committing to change

RESULTS often become the goal, but what if you can't find the motivation to get started and get the results to make your routine stick?

It can be tough to find the motivation to exercise when we're feeling tired, busy or distracted by other things. But what if we shift our focus away from the results and instead aim to find motivation through creating positive habits and achievable change?

By making small, positive changes and committing to them, we can slowly build a habit of consistent exercise. With consistency, we'll begin to see and feel changes in our well-being, though it may take 3–4 months to feel a significant change in strength, endurance, sleep, energy, confidence and overall health, especially if you want it to be sustainable and achievable for life. Once we experience these changes though, we'll naturally feel more motivated to continue on our journey towards better health.

For many of us, if we don't feel or see immediate improvements, we can become demotivated. You must allow time. Your future health is not seasonal, it is a daily work in progress and will continue to be.

Everyone is different, but 30 days can be long enough to help you create a new habit, and this is why the 30-Day Plan will be instrumental in helping you create change or continue on from where you are.

How to get results from the 30-Day Plan

- You need to understand that getting results isn't just about movement. The type of movement you do matters alongside a balanced, healthy diet and your overall daily activity.
- Start noticing how it makes you feel. Are you feeling more energised? Perhaps you are sleeping better or feeling calmer. How do you feel after you have done the exercise? Write it down and when you find yourself making excuses, you can remind yourself about why you are doing this and how amazing you will feel.
- Be kind to yourself. Don't beat yourself up or feel like there's no point if progress is slow. Slow equals sustainable, so keep going.
- Sleep (see Chapter 14), rest and recovery are integral parts of this plan and ones that can be overlooked or dismissed as contributing factors if you are not starting to sleep or feel better.
- Undereating and undernourishment of our changing body is another hurdle that many women going through menopause face. These can hinder you from getting the results you want.

Getting started

Starting and committing to an exercise routine can be challenging, especially if you're experiencing severe perimenopausal symptoms. It can also be confusing to determine the best way to move during this time, which can make it even harder to create a fitter, calmer and stronger life. It's crucial to acknowledge these obstacles and take action towards your fitness goals.

So how do we start and stick?

Find your WHY

If you are looking for a quick fix or a shortcut, you may start but you will not get the desired results in the long run. So, before you start the most important thing is to find your WHY:

- Have you been struggling with self-confidence and anxiety?

- Have you been experiencing more aches and pains?

- Would you like to have more energy?

- Would you like to sleep better?

- Would you like to feel less out of breath after climbing the stairs?

- Do you want to be strong and mobile enough to run around after your family?

- Do you just want to feel better?

If you have answered YES to one or more of the above, then use those as your WHY.

Knowing your why will help you work out why you want to exercise. It encourages you to search inwards and put the purpose before your goal. It gives you an opportunity to take ownership of your health and well-being and set about discovering your true needs at this time.

As an example, my why is to ensure I build a strong, resilient body so I can optimise my future health and stay active and mobile for years to come.

Self-sabotage

Much of sticking to a plan, whether it's eating or exercise, is about balance and making it fun so you can stick with it. If you go out one night and make food choices that might not be the best, that's OK. Don't be tempted to hit the 'sod it' button. And if you miss an exercise session one day, don't be tempted to give up on your eating plan too. Cut yourself some slack and try to get back on course the next day.

We convince ourselves that it has all gone to pot, and then we think we're back to square one. That couldn't be further from the truth.

In those situations, what I would love to encourage you to do is just to stop and recognise what you've done is OK. Have fun. Park it.

If it's not a daily choice and it happens occasionally, it won't affect anything. Enjoy that moment rather than feeling guilty about it. Move on to the next day and return to making those sensible choices you set yourself for the rest of the week.

Exercise after surgery

If you have had a surgical menopause, you must follow your doctor's advice when it comes to getting started or getting back into exercise. Much will depend on the type of surgery you had, but please note the following:

Walking is always a first choice and when you have had the all-clear that your wounds have healed, you may be allowed to swim.

DO NOT lift any heavy objects during your recovery and until you have been given the go-ahead from someone who is medically trained to authorise this.

Most advice is that you can start or resume gentle exercise 6–8 weeks after surgery, but this will vary from person to person. Your complete recovery time from a hysterectomy/mastectomy is usually 3 months to heal from the inside out, but as with all these things please make sure you have had clearance from your GP.

The 30-Day Plan in this book is only suitable once you have had a full recovery and have completed a full assessment from your GP that you can take part in this type of exercise programme.

CHAPTER 8

Types of Movement

Being able to move and ageing is a privilege denied to many. Your body is fantastic, and it deserves the chance to be strong so it can enable you to continue to do all the things you hope to do well into later life.

For the last 30 years, there has been a significant increase in the lifespan of women. In 1951, the life expectancy of females in the UK at birth was 80.7. However, as of 2020, this number has risen to 90.2.[21] This data is crucial in guiding us on how to maintain a healthy lifestyle before, during and after menopause.

Movement is the key component to the 30-Day Plan and it's important to know that diet alone will not help you build muscle or future-proof your body. I have put the plan together by incorporating many of the most beneficial exercises that mimic everyday movement, so that you can ensure this next chapter of your life is lived well and in good health. When it comes to movement, you must look at making long-term achievable and sustainable changes and adding strength training and weights to your routine. Remember, your body is not seasonal and needs to be moved and nourished 365 days of the year.

We have looked at the benefits of movement, so here we will unravel some myths and look at what we need to do to build a fitter, calmer, stronger body. How we move our bodies and the movements we choose to do all have different outcomes. They can be done alone or together as part of the programme and will all complement each other and the strength training exercises.

What we know is that you need to get your heart rate up (see page 73) to make sure you are giving your future self the best possible opportunity to stay fit and healthy. It is recommended that you aim for 150 minutes a week, unless you have been advised otherwise by your doctor. I like to break this down to 30 minutes a day, 5 days a week so it seems more achievable.[22] Even if you are at home with limited equipment, you can still do plenty of things to achieve this.

Did you know that according to the Centers for Disease Control and Prevention, gardening qualifies as exercise? Getting outside in the garden for 30–45 minutes can burn up to 300 calories and elevate your heart rate. It will also increase your endorphins, the feel-good hormones, and can increase your mobility.[23]

Walking is one of the most underrated ways of moving our bodies. If you can try to get outside for 20 minutes a day and walk at a good pace, you will reap the benefits and feel improvements in your overall well-being within 4–6 weeks.

Cycling has to be one of the most enjoyable ways to get movement in and something the whole family can be involved with. Pick a few routes with some hills to get the heart rate up and remember to remind yourself and any moaning family members that what goes up, must come down.

Even housework, which in my opinion has to be one of the least enjoyable ways to get movement in, can be a great all-over body workout. Bending and twisting will allow your body to work through a number of planes and will help with balance and mobility. Just make sure when you are picking things up to bend at the knees and avoid putting too much pressure on your lower back.

There are so many ways to move your body that don't involve hefty gym memberships. Finding movement you love will empower and motivate you to think about future-proofing your body for mobility, strength, and longevity, giving you energy for life.

Measuring your heart rate

A major benefit to moving is that you will increase your heart rate.

Your heart is like any other muscle and needs physical activity to keep it healthy. Getting your heart to beat faster will train your body to move oxygen and blood to your muscles more efficiently.

You may have a fitness tracker or want to invest in one so you can monitor your heart rate and other statistics, which is fine if you feel this would help you stay accountable, but please err on the side of caution in terms of it being 100 per cent accurate. I am also determined to encourage you to move based on how it makes you feel and not by consistently striving for numbers, be that on a watch or the bathroom scales.

I have included this table so you can monitor your efforts regardless of technology and base your session on moving more intuitively. Before technology advanced, most people measured their efforts using the RPE (rate of perceived exertion) scale.

The RPE scale measures the intensity of your exercise, with the scale running from 0–10. The numbers relate to how easy or difficult you find an activity. For example, 0 (nothing at all) would be how you feel when sitting in a chair; 10 (very, very heavy) is how you feel at the end of an exercise stress test or after a challenging activity.

You should exercise at a level somewhere between 3 (moderate) and 4 (somewhat heavy). When using this rating scale, remember to include feelings of shortness of breath and how tired you feel.

You can use this scale for all types of workouts, including running, and it's a great way to start understanding your body and feeling what it needs rather than forcing it to do something that will only make you want to quit or leave you feeling unsatisfied.

RPE CHART RATE OF PERCEIVED EXERTION

This chart is used to measure the intensity of each movement using a scale of 1-10.

10	COULD NOT PERFORM MORE REPS OR ADD WEIGHT
9.5	COULD NOT DO MORE REPS, BUT COULD ADD SLIGHTLY MORE WEIGHT
9	COULD DO 1 MORE REP
8.5	COULD DEFINITELY DO 1 MORE REP, POSSIBLY 2
8	COULD DO 2 MORE REPS
7.5	COULD DEFINITELY DO 2 MORE REPS, POSSIBLY 3
7	COULD DO 3 MORE REPS
5-6	COULD DO 4-6 MORE REPS
1-4	VERY LIGHT, LITTLE TO NO EFFORT

What is the best way to move during menopause?

The best way in reality is any way. Movement is absolutely critical and this is what I would love you to take away, but if you want to optimise your potential and give yourself the best chance of staying strong and mobile as you age, then lifting weights really is the best.

Finding a love of lifting weights when I was in the full grips of my perimenopause was life-changing. Many women can't determine why they are losing muscle or suffering from joint aches and pains, restricting their mobility. Lifting weights can help alleviate these symptoms, not exacerbate them.

Cardio versus weights

Cardio is any activity that raises your heart rate and breathing. Our muscles need oxygen to function and when we challenge them for a period of time, we will breathe faster as we need to get oxygen out to the muscles.

Lifting weights repeatedly requires much more work from your muscles so they will need more oxygen. As with cardio, we start breathing faster so our heart starts pumping faster.

Lifting weights is cardio but that doesn't negate the fact that running, cycling and the traditional forms of cardio sit nicely alongside and are also an important of your ongoing plan.

Of course, there are a number of other ways to move during menopause as you will see later on.

Functional movement

In this programme, we will be using movements that mimic day-to-day movements, or functional moves as they are better known in the industry. They are functional because they help your body move safely in your everyday life.

We can incorporate functional movements into our exercise routine and by also adding weights, we are building total-body strength, power, stamina and future-proofing our health.

There are seven basic movements the human body can perform, and all other exercises are merely variations of these seven: Squat, Lunge, Push, Pull, Bend/Hinge, Twist/Rotation and Gait. When performing all these movements, you will be able to stimulate all of the major muscle groups in your body. We should try to include all seven basic movements in our workouts.

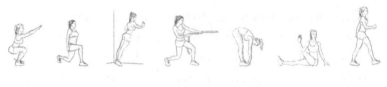

squat   lunge   push   pull   bend   twist   gait

- **Squat**

The squat is one of the most complex movements the body can do. It's considered important as part of our day-to-day life because the simple squat is comparable to sitting down and standing up. The muscles targeted are your glutes, core and quads.

- **Lunge**

Lunges help lower body strength and stability. Many women feel off balance when they perform this move as their body is at a disadvantaged stance, as you put one foot in front of the other. This move requires stability and balance, and this is something many woman notice. Instead of avoiding this pattern we need to practise to help build mobility. The lunge is a vital movement pattern that transfers well into walking, stair climbing and picking things up from the floor. Lunges will challenge your glutes, quads, core and hamstrings.

- **Push**

The push motion involves pushing something away from your body; this movement requires core and lower body stability. You may be wondering why we need to focus on that movement pattern. Without realising it, you push yourself out of chairs and push doors open; all require strength in your chest, triceps and shoulders.

- **Pull**

The pulling motion consists of pulling something towards your body. We may pull shopping bags over our shoulders, pull a car door shut or reach for things up high out of the cupboard. This requires us to have strength in our shoulders, chest, back and core.

- **Bend/Hinge**

Every day we find ourselves bending over to pick things up. Many women I see complain of lower back pain and this is often due to a weak posterior chain. When we talk about the posterior chain we are referring to your hamstrings, glutes and lower back. So, we must focus on exercises that will help us strengthen this area. Making sure that we are bending down properly and have the strength to be able to do so is important when it comes to the hinge movement. It is one of the most functional daily movements.

- **Twist/Rotation**

All too often, we move more frequently in one plane. What I mean is we usually find ourselves getting up or down, moving forwards or backwards and from side to side. The twisting or rotation movement is not something we often focus on, yet I see that it can cause many problems. Your core and obliques play a huge role in creating balance and stability. Being able to move in every direction can help prevent injuries.

- **Gait**

The ability to walk is a basic part of daily life and should be a priority and focus in any training programme. While this may seem obvious, it is an excellent way to start and get movement in, especially if you are a beginner. Your gait is a combination of multiple movements.

Strength training

I want to encourage every woman from the age of 35 to start thinking about preparing for the next stage of life by adding weights to their exercise regime if they haven't already. This is the only way, alongside a protein-rich diet, that you'll build muscle.

It is never too late to start and, by doing so, you will strengthen your bones, build muscle, manage many other symptoms of menopause and give yourself the best opportunity to age well.

Did you know you have 650 skeletal muscles in your body, which contract when they receive signals from motor neurons? Motor neurons tell your muscles to contract, and the more frequently your muscles receive those signals, the stronger you get.[24] So, the phrase 'use it or lose it' very much comes into play when it comes to building muscle.

I speak to and coach thousands of women who are concerned that they will bulk up when they lift weights, but I can assure you this won't happen.

What's happening when we lift weights and why is it so important in building muscle?

When we place our muscles under pressure from lifting, we cause tiny tears in our tissue. The size of the tear will depend on the amount of exertion you put the muscle under.[25] If you have a particularly challenging session, you will most likely have sore muscles after training, known as DOMS (delayed onset muscle soreness).

Allow time for rest and recovery, as it is the muscle tissue repairs that build stronger, leaner muscle. While this sounds a little odd, these little tears contribute to muscle growth.

As your body rebuilds that muscle, it increases the muscle size, strength and capacity. This kind of training will help combat the age-related muscle loss that I keep talking about. Strength training will also help with heart, joint and bone health and offset the decline of bone mineral density and prevent osteoporosis. In addition, it can help reduce body fat and increase the ability to burn calories more efficiently.

What weights to use

You can add weights or resistance to your training in many ways. It is sensible to begin with body weight and progress slowly.

• **Body weight**
You can do many exercises with little or no equipment. Try press ups, pull ups, planks, lunges and squats.

• **Resistance bands**
Resistance bands are inexpensive. You can choose from many resistance levels and types in nearly any sports shop or online.

• **Free weights**
Barbells and dumbbells are great strength-training tools, but can be costly. If you don't have weights at home, you can use cans or wine bottles. This will restrict you on how heavy you can lift though, so investing in some weights is a great idea.

• **Weight machines**
Most fitness centres offer various resistance machines.

How heavy?
High weights, low reps
Lifting heavier weights with low repetitions will create muscle mass and overall strength. It will also allow you to challenge your muscles more. It is more time efficient and will build more bone density, which is essential at this time.

HIIT

High-intensity interval training has gained much attention in the last few years.

It is a quick and effective method but it comes with risks. Don't get me wrong, HIIT workouts are an excellent way to get your exercise done and dusted in a shorter amount of time, and if it's something you are used to, then that's OK, to an extent. But when you aren't sleeping well during menopause, these types of workouts can send you into 'over-training mode'.

As we go through menopause, our bodies undergo significant changes, particularly with our hormones, which can put enormous stress on our bodies.

Here's the thing – if we are doing the wrong workouts and not sleeping well during menopause, then we can't recover from the training. And not all exercise classes are designed for healthy ageing or take into account a woman with declining oestrogen. I have seen so many exhausted women whose joints are hurting and whose knees are aching.

HIIT and overtraining, coupled with lack of sleep, can lead to an increase in our stress hormone, cortisol. When cortisol stays high for too long, it interferes with our sleep hormone, melatonin, and our blood sugar hormone, insulin. When both insulin and cortisol remain higher than they should overnight, this not only interferes with our normal fat-burning mechanisms, but we also don't recover from our exercise. If you love HIIT and want to keep it as part of the programme, I recommend you limit your sessions to twice a week.

LISS

Low-intensity steady-state cardio has many health benefits, including improved blood flow, reduced stress, lower risk of heart disease and improved brain function. It is easier to do and gentler on the body than HIIT and it's appropriate for beginners.

When doing LISS cardio, the goal is to keep your heart rate at around 50–65 per cent of your maximum heart rate.

LISS is the opposite of HIIT and is associated with running, cycling, brisk walking and swimming, which entail longer sessions of low-intensity intervals. It is kinder on your bones and joints, so for anyone suffering from aches and pains, this would be a great way to move until you have built up more strength and feel comfortable and confident to move on to something more challenging.

However, if your goal is weight loss, LISS training requires extended periods of training time, which can be a challenge for a busy lifestyle.

Pilates

Chloe Hodgson, an expert in this field and founder of Chloe's Pilates, says Pilates is an excellent exercise choice for women navigating the challenges of menopause. It helps restore calm, improve balance and build and tone your muscles. It also supports bone health and may help to prevent osteoporosis.

We all want a long life and know that we need to be as fit as possible in order to be able to enjoy our later years independently and in good health.

Joseph Pilates cleverly formed his exercise method to be as beneficial for the mind as it is for the body. His exercises are rooted in the principles of concentration, control, centring, precision, breathing and flow. As Joseph Pilates himself stated: 'Pilates is the mastery of your mind gaining complete control over your body. You're only as old as your spine. The mind, when housed within a healthful body, possesses a glorious sense of power.'

Here are seven convincing benefits that Pilates offers women in midlife:

1. Pilates improves both your strength and flexibility while increasing joint mobility.
2. Pilates exercises are slow, controlled movements, making it a low-impact option suitable for various fitness levels.
3. Pilates exercises can be modified and adapted to meet your individual needs and fitness goals.
4. Pilates breathing improves core muscle function, promotes mindfulness, reduces stress, and develops movement precision.
5. Pilates helps to strengthen your back muscles and abdominals, which will not only help with back pain but also improve your posture.
6. Pilates complements strength training sessions by promoting core strength, muscle balance, flexibility, mobility and improved posture, leading to more effective and well-rounded fitness.
7. In Pilates, we move through all our joints, keeping them supple and mobile despite the hormonal changes our bodies are going through.

Yoga

Yoga is an excellent way of managing and reducing stress as we go through menopause. It can immediately begin to reduce the stress and overproduction of cortisol, enabling your body to function better, and you to think more clearly and help remain mentally and physically strong.

Yoga also helps maintain your physical strength and keeps your body flexible. Yoga is renowned for helping the mind, which, as we know, can become more anxious through menopause and midlife. As meditation is a part of yoga practice and mindfulness helps a great deal in managing anxiety, if you haven't tried yoga, you most definitely should.

We know that postmenopausal women are more susceptible to heart disease and Type 2 diabetes; if movement has become a thing of the past, yoga would be a great way to start getting your body moving. Yoga can be maintained well into your 80s or even 90s as it is a low-impact, weight-bearing activity.

Dance

The moves used in dance, especially ballroom and Latin dancing, are great exercises for bone health because dance is a weight-bearing exercise, which is good for bone density, improves balance and works on our body awareness skills, which can help prevent falls as we age.

Walking

This underrated, overlooked, yet easily accessible form of exercise can be so beneficial and is an all-over body workout. Walking is free and relatively simple and is one of the easiest ways to start moving your body if you are new to exercise.

You do not have to walk for hours. A brisk 10-minute daily walk has many health benefits and counts towards your 150 minutes of weekly exercise, as recommended in the physical activity guidelines for adults aged 19 to 64.[26]

If you have not been active for a while, gradually build your walk from 10 minutes one week to 20 the next and try to go at a faster pace to feel the benefits. Walking is beneficial, but it is also getting outside that significantly impacts your mental well-being. Being in nature can be such a positive experience.

You could incorporate walking into your daily routine by allowing time to get to a destination and hopping off the bus or tube a few stops before. It can also be an excellent opportunity to listen to a podcast or call friends for a catch-up.

Running

Running, like walking, is free and available to most of us. While it has many benefits, I would encourage any woman in menopause to ensure they warm up and cool down properly to avoid injury at this time.

I also think we must remember how hard running can be on our joints, and if you are new to the sport, please don't try to go from 0–5K in a short time. Not only will you leave yourself open to injury, but you will likely put yourself off trying again, having put unrealistic expectations on yourself.

If you have been running for a long time and are finding it harder, don't be disheartened. Take a step back and, if you haven't already, try to add some strength training sessions to your weekly programme. This will positively affect your overall health, and you may find it helps your stamina and endurance.

Cycling

Being outside has so many positive effects on our overall well-being. Like walking and running, cycling is a simple way to get the heart pumping and body moving and something that the whole family can do together, which, if you are stretched for time on the weekends, can be a great activity. It is also kinder on your joints and can be a fun way to get some movement in on holiday.

Swimming

Swimming is an excellent way to work your entire body and cardiovascular system. An hour of swimming burns almost as many calories as running without all the impact on your bones and joints.

Swimming works your entire body. It can increase your heart rate without stressing your body, tones muscles and builds strength and endurance. It's brilliant for those suffering joint aches and pains and is a great mood booster.

It's also another great family activity and you can start at any level and age.

Spin

This can elevate your heart rate, which is beneficial, but it can have the same effect as cortisol if done too often, so be mindful of the number of sessions you do in your week and make sure that you are also adding some strength sessions in.

Spin is a great workout and, again, it is kinder on the joints and can be a good way to meet people or encourage friends to join you as you cycle to loud music, often feeling euphoric for hours after.

Barre

Barre classes combine low-impact exercises like stretching or upper arm circles with faster-paced physical activity, such as jumping squats, to create a variety of aerobic conditioning sessions, which have been shown over time to be more effective at improving core strength than traditional sit ups can offer alone.

Barre classes significantly improve your mind–body connection, balance, stability and strength to relieve aches and pains often experienced among those experiencing perimenopause. Classes are low-impact but high-intensity and allow you to build strength kindly for your body. Your joints (and your pelvic floor) will thank you.

Barre doesn't just exercise our bodies, it also works our brains! This workout keeps our cognitive skills sharp with directional changes and listening to and following instructions.

Types of movement

Strength training is always a non-negotiable, but I also want you to understand the benefits of other movements, so that when you move on after the 30-Day Plan you are equipped with the knowledge of what will work for you, and you can continue to make progress.

We should aim to move in some way daily as it helps with overall health and well-being, boosts mood, improves heart health, helps regulate blood sugar, reduces blood pressure, uses calories and helps with mobility. TDEE (see page 92) is affected by daily movement and for many, it can be the piece of the puzzle that is missing in making progress. Be sure to note if weight loss or management is one of your goals.

Types of movement	Benefits	To note
Strength training	• Builds and maintains muscle mass • Strengthens bones • Helps joint flexibility • Creates mobility • Builds self-confidence • Helps regulate blood sugar • Decreases risk of falls • Lowers risk of injury • Improves heart health • Boosts mood • Improves brain health • Lowers the risk of high blood pressure • Suitable for all levels and ages • Boosts immune system	Start gradually and always make sure you are aware of your form in order to avoid injury. Invest in some good sturdy dumbbells. Warm up and cool down. Allow time in between your sessions so your muscles can repair.
HIIT	• Quick • Improves stamina • Can increase strength • Good for your heart • Helps regulate blood sugar • Lowers the risk of high blood pressure • Boosts mood	Too much HIIT can elevate your cortisol levels, which can have a negative impact on a menopausal woman. I suggest 1–2 sessions a week MAX.
LISS	• Suitable for all levels • Lowers the risk of high blood pressure • Kinder on joints • Good for endurance • Good for a recovery session • Boosts mood • Boosts immune system	LISS is great but it does require more time – (45–60 minutes). It's great if you are doing endurance events. You can get bored, so mix up your LISS with walking, cycling, swimming and jogging.

Pilates	• Helps relieve tension • Promotes body awareness • Kinder on joints • Builds muscle, balance, stability and mobility • Improves flexibility • Increases core strength • Decreases back pain • Improves posture • Suitable for all levels and ages • Boosts mood • Boosts immune system	Pilates is a great addition to a programme as we go through menopause and midlife. It will help with recovery and can be a wonderful option for many who are experiencing joint aches and pains.
Yoga	• Helps relieve tension • Improves breathing • Kinder on joints • Builds muscle, balance, stability and mobility • Improves flexibility • Increases core strength • Decreases back pain • Improves posture • Suitable for all levels and ages • Boosts mood • Boosts immune system	Yoga is a great addition to a programme as we go through menopause and midlife. It will help with recovery and can be a wonderful option for many who are experiencing joint aches and pains. It can help you to focus more on your breath, which can benefit overall health and well-being.

Dance	• Improves heart health • Can help with strength and endurance • Increases your aerobic fitness • Helps with coordination, agility and flexibility • Music can help with mood • It can be free • Suitable for all levels and ages • Boosts immune system	Going to a dance class, dancing at home or on a night out is a mood-booster and can build self-confidence.
Walking	• Suitable for all levels and ages • For all the family • Lowers the risk of high blood pressure • Kinder on joints • Good for endurance • Good for a recovery session • Great for your mental health • It's free • Readily possible • Boosts mood • Boosts immune system	It is really important to ensure you add some strength training sessions alongside your walks to get the maximum benefits of your fitness plan.
Running	• It can help manage stress • It's free • Suitable for all ages and levels • Great for heart and lung health • Helps regulate blood sugar • Boosts mood • Boosts immune system	Incorporate strength training alongside your running, especially to help with recovery and endurance. If you are experiencing aches and pains, it's okay to rest and recover and come back to running when you are up for the challenge.

Cycling	• It can help manage stress • It's free • Kinder on joints • Good for endurance • Suitable for all ages and levels and a great family activity • Great for heart and lung health • Helps balance sugar levels • Boosts mood • Boosts immune system	Incorporate strength training alongside your cycling, especially to help with endurance and balance.
Spin	• Kinder on joints • Good for endurance	Be mindful of the amount you do as it can raise cortisol levels. Spin is a great way to meet people and the music can really boost your endorphins.
Barre	• Helps relieve tension • Promotes body awareness • Kinder on joints • Builds muscle, balance, stability and mobility • Improves flexibility • Increases core strength • Decreases back pain • Improves posture • Suitable for all levels and ages • Boosts mood • Boosts immune system	You will most likely need to invest in some bands, low weights and have a stable chair to perform some of the moves.

Exercise snacks

These are short bursts of exercise, for example doing jumping jacks whilst waiting for the kettle to boil, or standing on one foot whilst queuing. It would be wrong to assume that this easy way of exercising is suitable for a long period of time. It's a great way to get movement in on time-poor days and a wonderful way to build confidence if you are starting, but it will not be as beneficial as setting aside allocated workout time.

- If you have no time something is better than nothing
- Good to build up from scratch
- Can be done anywhere
- Boosts mood
- Boosts confidence

Weight loss and movement

Weight loss should not be your sole and only focus when choosing what movement to incorporate into your programme, but I have to be realistic and address the fact that many women would like sensible guidance on how to lose unwanted weight for good.

Exercise, and strength training in particular, can help you maintain and lose weight but you must also look at your daily activity. You will need to see what you put in versus what you put out in order for weight loss to happen.

In order for weight loss to be sustainable, you must understand it takes time, just like building muscle. Taking shortcuts can hinder it being a lifelong change. The 30-Day Plan is a great example of how we can combine all this for lifelong sustainable change.

For many women going through menopause, sudden weight

gain is a huge concern with many not understanding why this has happened and why it is they are not losing weight based on the exercise they are doing.

How you move throughout your day plays a key role here. While I don't want us to get hung up on calories, we must understand how they are needed for our bodies to carry out many daily functions, not just exercise.

The importance of TDEE (total daily exercise expenditure)

TDEE[27] stands for *Total Daily Energy Expenditure* and is the total number of calories you burn in a given day. Four key factors determine your TDEE:

- Basal Metabolic Rate (BMR)

- Thermic Effect of Activity (TEA)

- Non-Exercise Activity Thermogenesis (NEAT)

- Thermic Effect of Food (TEF)

Basal Metabolic Rate (BMR)

This refers to the number of calories your body burns each day to keep you alive. BMR does not include physical activity, the process of digestion or things like walking from one room to another.

BMR is the number of calories your body would expend in a 24-hour period if all you did was lie in bed all day long. This is the absolute bare minimum of calories to ensure your survival.

Thermic Effect of Activity (TEA)

Thermic Effect of Activity is the number of calories burned due to exercise and planned physical activity.

The thermic effect of exercise is highly variable from one person to another or even from one day to another for the same person, as the intensity of training, length of the workout and training frequency all impact your weekly thermic effect of activity.

Non-Exercise Activity Thermogenesis (NEAT)

Non-exercise Activity Thermogenesis (NEAT) is the number of calories expended during daily movement that is not categorised as structured exercise.

NEAT includes activities such as walking the dog, moving from one room to another or taking the stairs to your office. It plays a valuable role and is the reason I include 8,000–10,000 steps a day in the plan. You need to ensure you move during the day in order to optimise your progress.

NEAT is highly variable from one person to another and can play a rather large or small role in your overall TDEE, depending on how physically active your job or daily happenings are.

Thermic Effect of Food (TEF)

When we eat food, our body must expend energy to digest the food. This energy expenditure is referred to as the Thermic Effect of Food. It involves breaking down the protein, carbohydrates and fat you consume into individual amino acids, sugars and fatty acids that are then absorbed and used by the body to carry out all of its processes, including (but not limited to) building new tissue, synthesising hormones and producing neurotransmitters.

The Thermic Effect of Food generally accounts for 10 per cent of your total daily energy expenditure but can be slightly higher or lower based on the exact macronutrient composition of your diet.[28]

For example, protein requires more energy to digest than carbohydrates or fat. So, if you're eating a high-protein diet, you will burn more calories, slightly, than if you were to eat the same number of calories but with a significantly lower amount of protein.

Summary

- With little understanding of how our declining hormones impact us at this time, many women over-exercise and under-eat, which can harm our hormone health and fitness journeys.

- Movement through menopause is important for more than just the aesthetics.

- Exercise will help manage many of your menopausal symptoms. It will also help you find mental and physical strength you didn't know you had. This can be empowering when you are presented with a myriad of symptoms.

- We need to think about exercise at this time of life as being primarily for our heart, bones, muscles, joints and brain, not simply as a way of managing weight, which I know is high on the list of priorities for many women.

- Adding strength training is an absolute non-negotiable if you want to build a fitter, calmer, stronger body for life.

PART 3

This is Your Fitter, Calmer, Stronger in 30 Days Plan

One Day or Day One. You Decide.

Paul Coelho

This is where you are going to commit and make change happen to future-proof your body. You bought this book for a reason and I am guessing the 30-Day Plan was a huge part of investing in yourself. Please make sure you have read through all the sections and the plans so you can see what is involved.

The 30-Day Plan is a detailed tried-and-tested programme

that will make you feel stronger. For some you may well notice change quickly, but it is important to remember that real change can take 3–4 months.

You can access the plan via the QR code on page 97 so that you can do the workouts in real time and feel like you are part of a class, which will help motivate you. If you don't have access, all the plans and exercises are explained and illustrated in the coming pages.

Please note that this plan is not centred around temporary solutions or flashy trends. Instead, it aims to guide you towards gradual, realistic adjustments that will ultimately result in a stronger, more serene, healthier version of yourself that can be maintained for life.

CHAPTER 9

Set Yourself Up For Success

I have created two 30-Day Plans because we must be realistic that everyone will have a different entry level and starting point.

This section will give you all the tips you need to get started with the right mindset and encourage you to track your progress realistically so this becomes achievable and sustainable.

The beginner's guide will give you the confidence you need to progress onto the intermediate guide. The intermediate guide is for people who have a good level of fitness and experience lifting weights. They will also have good form and be ready to push themselves harder. Please do not jump to the intermediate level if you are new to exercise.

What you need to start

- **Equipment**

Please make sure you have a set of 3kg and 5kg dumbbells for the BEGINNERS plan as this programme looks at encouraging you to get lifting weights so you can feel the benefits of the things we have talked about.

I would suggest you look at anything between 5kg and 10kg for the INTERMEDIATE/ADVANCED plan.

- **A mat**

This will help protect your back when we do some of the abdominal exercises and it will provide a good base under you for stability– carpets and wooden floors will be too slippery and could lead to injury.

- **A water bottle**

It is important to stay hydrated through your sessions, so always ensure you have enough water to hand so your workout isn't interrupted.

- **Comfortable clothes to work out in**

These are essential. You don't have to have a gym kit, you just need something light and comfortable. I would recommend you wear a supportive sports bra or similar as it is important to make sure you feel supported across the chest area, especially for ladies who have larger chests. If you are uncomfortable or feel unsupported, this can really put you off.

- **Trainers**

I train in bare feet to ensure my feet are grounded and stable. You can choose to wear trainers if you like – this is a personal preference.

- **A notebook**

Start journalling your fitness progress and noting the tweaks you have made. This will help you keep note of the improvements you are feeling, allowing the programme to be more motivating.

Three important points to help you succeed

- Preparing for each week and following the 30-Day Plan and menu ideas will help you reach your full potential.
- Make sure to set clear intentions for the 30 days and focus on achieving your goals every morning.
- Remember, this lifestyle is achievable if you commit to bringing about positive change in 30 days.

Tips to set yourself up for success

- Forgive yourself if you are not up for the challenge on a particular day; just try not to miss more than 2 days in a row.

- Follow the fitness programme – don't try to jump ahead. This is about making slow and sustainable changes.

- Try to get 8,000–10,000 steps in a day on top of your sessions, as all daily activity will help you progress further.

- Warming up, cooling down and rest days are important. In the plan, the stretch & mobility days are rest days, as are the Sunday mindfulness sessions.

- Eating nourishing, balanced meals is fundamental for success.

- Make notes on how you feel. Don't look for results immediately – FEEL THEM.

- If you are struggling, have a little rest and come back to a session later in the day. If you need to break up the sessions, that is okay. Progress will be seen when you don't feel the need to break them up – this is a positive thing to note and feel.

- Allow time for the sessions. They have a rough time guide on them, so you will know if you are able to complete them in the time you have allocated yourself.

- Try to get your workout done in the morning. If this means getting up 30 minutes earlier, please try to do this. It's not that it's a better time, but you will find you have more energy for the rest of the day and the evening often doesn't allow us the time.

- Hold yourself accountable by telling your family or friends that you are committing to future-proofing your body and that you'd love their support, especially over the 30 days, so that you can give it your best shot.

- Prioritise sleep.

- Avoid alcohol (if you really can't, then 1–2 glasses a week MAX).

- Let me know how you are feeling – I'd love to hear from you. If you have any questions, email fittercalmerstrongerin30days@ gmail.com

> *I'm grateful for the encouragement that came with this plan to get back to exercise being a routine and part of my day. I'm doing 3 strength workouts a week now too. The plan has set me up with good habits. I already feel so much fitter and stronger.*
>
> **Lynn**

Tracking your progress

Please remember that there are many different contributing factors to how a workout session may unfold on the day. Your symptoms (see Chapter 2) and where you are in your cycle (see Chapter 4) will have a significant impact on your sessions.

Try to track and work out why it might be you aren't feeling up for the challenge so you can build a pattern and not only understand why your body isn't responding on that day but, more importantly, you know you aren't going backwards and you can forgive yourself. Remember, you aren't going to feel changes overnight and each week you may feel something different.

See the table overleaf as an example of things you could look to note that will encourage you to stick to the programme. Use a scoring system of 1–10 to see the progress, where 1 is the lowest and 10 is the best, and fill in the table after your sessions. Add more columns as you begin to feel different changes.

	Increased Energy	Better Sleep	More Confidence	Improved Anxiety	Aches & Pains	Better Mood	Fitter	Calmer	Motivated
Days 1–7	2	1	2	2	1	3	n/a	n/a	n/a
Days 8–14 THIS WEEK MAY FEEL HARD – DON'T QUIT!	3	3	4	4	2	4	3	n/a	n/a
Days 15–21 CHANGE IS HAPPENING – YOU ARE DOING THIS!	5	5	5	6	5	6	5	6	n/a
Days 22–30	7	7	7	7	7	7	7	8	9

HOW THE PLAN WORKS

I have created two 30-day plans, one to cater for beginners and an intermediate plan for those who may already have a good fitness level but have plateaued and want to learn how they can make changes to continue to build strength or perhaps even lose a little bit of weight.

When we start incorporating weights in the beginner's plan, I will ask you to begin with lighter weights of 3kg and 5kg and to gradually build up. This approach ensures your muscles are ready to work with the pattern of movement and reduces the risk of injury.

If you already understand what you are doing and have a moderate level of fitness, the intermediate/advanced plan will aim to push you even harder so you can also see how to make progress at this time of life and how it is all possible and sustainable from home.

As I have mentioned, making changes can seem daunting, especially if you are experiencing some of the more crippling symptoms associated with menopause. Still, I hope this book will have given you the confidence and motivation to prioritise your long-term health and you are excited about the next steps you are taking in moving forward.

Regardless of your starting point, prepare for each week by writing down and making a note of your intentions. Follow the 30-Day Plan and menu ideas closely to optimise your well-being and make your intentions stick.

Before you start, take a PAR-Q+ test, which can be found online and is a 7-step questionnaire for use by persons of all ages.[29] It screens for evidence of risk factors during moderate physical activity and reviews the family history and disease severity.

If you answer yes to one or more questions, PLEASE consult a doctor about beginning physical activity.

Disclaimer

Please review the following before starting the 30-Day Plan.

Please note that this programme and the on-demand workouts have been designed to improve basic levels of fitness. It has not been designed for any specific issues that may be exacerbated by some of the more intense exercises.

Kate Rowe-Ham strongly recommends that you consult with your GP before beginning any exercise programme if you feel you have any pre-existing conditions. If you experience faintness, dizziness, pain or shortness of breath at any time while exercising, you should stop immediately. When participating in any exercise, there may be a possibility of physical injury.

If you engage in the 30-Day Plan, then you agree that you do so at your own risk, are voluntarily participating in these activities, assume all risk of injury to yourself, and agree to release and discharge Kate Rowe-Ham from any claims. This programme offers health, fitness, nutritional and menopause information and is designed for educational purposes only. You should not rely on this information as a substitute for professional medical advice. The use of any information provided is at your own risk.

Scanning the QR code on page 97 will enable you to create an account and have access to choose which 30-Day Plan you would like.

All the pre-recorded videos have been devised especially with you in mind.

CHAPTER 10

The Fitter, Calmer, Stronger in 30 Days Plan For Beginners

Before you start the plan make sure you have a set of dumbbells. Ideally you will look to be using 3kg and 5kg. You will need these ready for Week 2.

Days 1–7
You may notice a positive change in energy, sleep, confidence, anxiety etc. You are also likely to notice a few aches and pains as you embark on this new routine, but if they are not sharp or acute, they will ease as your body adapts.

Days 8–14
You may continue to feel similar benefits as on Days 1–7, but at the same time experience negative thoughts or a lull as the reality of making change begins to feel real. Look at the positive changes you have noted at this time and PUSH THROUGH (unless you have sharp or acute pains when exercising).

Days 15–28

You will really start to notice and feel how this programme is working and how this could change your life for good. Please keep making notes. The aches and pains may come and go, especially as we introduce longer workouts and potentially increase some of the weights. This is normal and is called DOMS (see page 205). You should now be thinking about how you want to continue and what elements you really want to stick to when it comes to moving forward.

Days 28–30

You will now have made some new habits that you want to keep and stick to because you can feel what a difference they have made. You are feeling FITTER, CALMER, STRONGER.

Don't think that this is it and you will go back to your old habits. This is really the beginning of a new journey. Look back over your notes and see how much you have progressed.

DAY 1	DAY 2	DAY 3	DAY 4	DAY 5	DAY 6	DAY 7
BODY-WEIGHT BASICS (15 MINS)	STRETCH & MOBILITY (15 MINS)	LOWER BODY BODY-WEIGHT (15 MINS)	ABS & CORE (15 MINS)	UPPER BODY BODY-WEIGHT (15 MINS)	STRETCH & MOBILITY (15 MINS)	FULL BODY (20 MINS)

DAY 8	DAY 9	DAY 10	DAY 11	DAY 12	DAY 13	DAY 14
UPPER BODY WEIGHTS (20 MINS)	BODY-WEIGHT BASICS (20 MINS)	ABS & CORE (15 MINS)	LOWER BODY WEIGHTS (20 MINS)	FULL BODY WEIGHTS (20 MINS	STRETCH & MOBILITY (15 MINS)	BREATH-WORK MEDIT-ATION

DAY 15	DAY 16	DAY 17	DAY 18	DAY 19	DAY 20	DAY 21
UPPER BODY (25 MINS)	BODY-WEIGHT BASICS (20 MINS)	STRETCH & MOBILITY (15 MINS)	UNILAT-ERAL LOWER BODY (25 MINS)	FULL BODY WEIGHTS (25 MINS	ABS & CORE (15 MINS)	BREATH-WORK MEDIT-ATION

DAY 22	DAY 23	DAY 24	DAY 25	DAY 26	DAY 27	DAY 28
UNILAT-ERAL UPPER BODY (35 MINS)	BODY-WEIGHT BASICS (25 MINS)	STRETCH & MOBILITY (15 MINS)	LOWER BODY WEIGHTS (30 MINS)	FULL BODY WEIGHTS (30 MINS)	STRETCH & MOBILITY (15 MINS)	BREATH-WORK MEDIT-ATION

DAY 29	DAY 30
ABS & CORE (15 MINS)	FULL BODY WEIGHTS (30 MINS)

Let's go!

DAYS 1–7: BACK TO BASICS WITH BODYWEIGHT

DAY 1	DAY 2	DAY 3	DAY 4	DAY 5	DAY 6	DAY 7
BODY-WEIGHT BASICS (15 MINS)	STRETCH & MOBILITY (15 MINS)	LOWER BODY BODY-WEIGHT (15 MINS)	ABS & CORE (15 MINS)	UPPER BODY BODY-WEIGHT (15 MINS)	STRETCH & MOBILITY (15 MINS)	FULL BODY (20 MINS)

You may be feeling slightly overwhelmed and anxious or worrying about how you are going to feel as you get ready to start. This is completely normal, and you are not alone. These first 7 days will allow your body to adapt to the new changes you are about to make.

We will also focus on your form, so you feel comfortable and confident as you move into Day 8 with a renewed sense of energy and excitement feeling the buzz from the last 7 days. Form is critical when it comes to avoiding injury, so the follow-along sessions will guide you on how to perform each move. If you can work out with access to a mirror, this will help you see that you are lifting correctly and safely.

It is normal to experience mild discomfort and some muscle soreness as you start, so don't let this put you off from continuing.

PLEASE ENSURE YOU WARM UP AND COOL DOWN BEFORE AND AFTER EACH SESSION

If you can't manage the full 45 seconds, don't worry. Do what you can and build up. It is about steady progress.

Don't forget to get your steps in on top of your workouts as part of your daily movement (TDEE).

Warm-up Routine	Time
Walkouts (page 184)	45 secs on / 15 secs rest
Wrist & Ankle Circles	45 secs on / 15 secs rest

Squats (page 160)	45 secs on / 15 secs rest
Release Press Ups (page 173)	45 secs on / 15 secs rest
Plank Rotations (page 170)	45 secs on / 15 secs rest
Star Steps/Jumps (page 193)	45 secs on / 15 secs rest

Cool-down Routine	Time
Piriformis Stretches (page 199)	45 secs on / 15 secs rest
Cat Cows (page 197)	45 secs on / 15 secs rest
Tricep Stretches (page 200)	45 secs on / 15 secs rest
The Baby (page 201)	45 secs on / 15 secs rest
Chest and Bicep Stretches (page 200)	45 secs on / 15 secs rest

Day 1 We are starting with a 15-minute beginners' bodyweight workout, so you can see how you can get a good workout in a short time, but also to allow you to get to grips with some of the principal and fundamental moves we will be using throughout the plan.

Bodyweight Basics			
	Round 1	Round 2	Round 3
Squats (page 160)	45 secs on 15 secs rest	45 secs on 15 secs rest	45 secs on 15 secs rest
Dead Bugs (page 182)	45 secs on 15 secs rest	45 secs on 15 secs rest	45 secs on 15 secs rest
Press Ups (page 172)	45 secs on 15 secs rest	45 secs on 15 secs rest	45 secs on 15 secs rest
Lateral Lunges (page 166)	45 secs on 15 secs rest	45 secs on 15 secs rest	45 secs on 15 secs rest
Walkouts (page 184)	45 secs on 15 secs rest	45 secs on 15 secs rest	45 secs on 15 secs rest

Day 2 This will stretch away some possible aches from Day 1. Please remember we are aiming for slow, sustainable change and progress.

Stretch & Mobility	Time / Reps / Rounds
Cat Cows (page 197)	x 5
Bird Dogs (page 197)	x 5 each side
Thread the Needles (page 198)	x 5 each side
Hip Flexors (page 199)	45 secs each side x 2
Piriformis Stretches (page 199)	45 secs each side x 2
	REPEAT x 2

Day 3 Focusing on the lower body and breaking up the body parts allows you an extra opportunity for recovery and means that you aren't aching all over.

Lower Body Bodyweight			
	Round 1	**Round 2**	**Round 3**
Squats (page 160)	45 secs on 15 secs rest	45 secs on 15 secs rest	45 secs on 15 secs rest
Aternating Reverse Lunges (page 162)	45 secs on 15 secs rest	45 secs on 15 secs rest	45 secs on 15 secs rest
Hip Thrusts (page 191)	45 secs on 15 secs rest	45 secs on 15 secs rest	45 secs on 15 secs rest
Good Mornings (page 172)	45 secs on 15 secs rest	45 secs on 15 secs rest	45 secs on 15 secs rest
Curtsy Lunges (page 165)	45 secs on 15 secs rest	45 secs on 15 secs rest	45 secs on 15 secs rest

Day 4 Focusing on building core strength in order to protect your lower back and work on the pelvic floor area.

Abs & Core			
	Round 1	**Round 2**	**Round 3**
Dead Bugs (page 182)	45 secs on 15 secs rest	45 secs on 15 secs rest	45 secs on 15 secs rest
Bikes (page 185)	45 secs on 15 secs rest	45 secs on 15 secs rest	45 secs on 15 secs rest
Plank Taps (page 183)	45 secs on 15 secs rest	45 secs on 15 secs rest	45 secs on 15 secs rest
Bird Dogs (page 197)	45 secs on 15 secs rest	45 secs on 15 secs rest	45 secs on 15 secs rest
Twists (page 186)	45 secs on 15 secs rest	45 secs on 15 secs rest	45 secs on 15 secs rest

Day 5 Focusing on the upper body and breaking up the body parts allows you an extra opportunity for recovery and means that you aren't aching all over.

Upper Body Bodyweight			
	Round 1	**Round 2**	**Round 3**
Walkouts (page 184)	45 secs on 15 secs rest	45 secs on 15 secs rest	45 secs on 15 secs rest
Bear Taps (page 192)	45 secs on 15 secs rest	45 secs on 15 secs rest	45 secs on 15 secs rest
Release Press Ups (page 173)	45 secs on 15 secs rest	45 secs on 15 secs rest	45 secs on 15 secs rest
Arm Circles (page 195)	45 secs on 15 secs rest	45 secs on 15 secs rest	45 secs on 15 secs rest
Punches (page 196)	45 secs on 15 secs rest	45 secs on 15 secs rest	45 secs on 15 secs rest

Day 6 Making sure we stretch out and mobilise is a fundamental part of the plan. We are looking to protect and strengthen our bodies, so making time for this is key and often means you will stick to the plan because you aren't overdoing your sessions or overloading your body.

Stretch & Mobility	Time / Reps / Rounds
Cat Cows (page 197)	x 5
Bird Dogs (page 197)	x 5 each side
Thread the Needles (page 198)	x 5 each side
Hip Flexors (page 199)	45 secs each side x 2
Piriformis Stretches (page 199)	45 secs each side x 2
	REPEAT x 2

Nearly finished Day 7 and I've gone from feeling embarrassed at how unfit I felt to now I am so proud I am doing the plan and doing something about it and I've survived the first 6 days. I am feeling the benefit of better food and three meals a day. I am feeling positive for all the new changes, and I am sure I can keep them up as they seem achievable.

Tina

Day 7 Finishing off the week positively with a longer all-over bodyweight workout.

Full Body			
	Round 1	**Round 2**	**Round 3**
Reverse Lunges Overhead (change sides halfway) (page 164)	45 secs on 15 secs rest	45 secs on 15 secs rest	45 secs on 15 secs rest
Squats (page 160)	45 secs on 15 secs rest	45 secs on 15 secs rest	45 secs on 15 secs rest
Plank Taps (page 183)	45 secs on 15 secs rest	45 secs on 15 secs rest	45 secs on 15 secs rest
Frog Pumps (page 167)	45 secs on 15 secs rest	45 secs on 15 secs rest	45 secs on 15 secs rest
Plank Rotations (page 170)	45 secs on 15 secs rest	45 secs on 15 secs rest	45 secs on 15 secs rest

DAYS 8–14: ADDING WEIGHTS TO YOUR WORKOUTS

DAY 8	DAY 9	DAY 10	DAY 11	DAY 12	DAY 13	DAY 14
UPPER BODY WEIGHTS (20 MINS)	BODY-WEIGHT BASICS (20 MINS)	ABS & CORE (15 MINS)	LOWER BODY WEIGHTS (20 MINS)	FULL BODY WEIGHTS (20 MINS)	STRETCH & MOBILITY (15 MINS)	BREATH-WORK MEDIT-ATION

Time to pick up those dumbbells you've invested in to help you build a fitter, calmer, stronger body.

These workouts will be broken down into sections, where we will repeat some of the moves for a number of repetitions. We will introduce these slowly and I would advise you to begin with the 3kg and see how they feel – keep the 5kg weights on standby.

You will be able to gauge if you are lifting heavy enough by how you feel. When you get to the last 2–3 reps (these are the last two or three repetitions) of the exercise we are performing, how does it feel – is it easy or does it feel tough?

For example, If the exercise is a squat and we are doing 12 reps or repetitions – are you finding it easy or hard as we get to the 12th one? If it is easy, this is an indication you should be lifting more weight. If you are struggling to finish, then this would indicate that you are lifting too heavy. If you find yourself struggling – it's OK. Complete the reps you can of that exercise and write it down – this is a great way to see progress because when you try again next week or in 2 weeks, you may be able to lift it. As I have said, this is about gradual progress.

Don't forget to get your daily steps in as well.

Day 8 We are doing a weighted upper body workout today. This will be 6 moves focusing on building strength in your arms, back, shoulders and core. You will need your 3kg weight for this.

Upper Body Weights			
Exercises – Set 1	**Round 1**	**Round 2**	**Round 3**
Bent Over Rows (page 174)	12–14 reps	10–12 reps	8–10 reps
Bent Arm Lateral Raises (page 176)	12–14 reps	10–12 reps	8–10 reps
Chest Presses (page 187)	12–14 reps	10–12 reps	8–10 reps
Exercises – Set 2	**Round 1**	**Round 2**	**Round 3**
Bicep Curls (page 176)	12–14 reps	10–12 reps	8–10 reps
Tricep Kickbacks (page 179)	12–14 reps	10–12 reps	8–10 reps
Overhead Presses (page 180)	12–14 reps	10–12 reps	8–10 reps

Day 9 Make sure you continue to build good habits by getting in some movement but going back to bodyweight for recovery.

Bodyweight Basics			
Exercises – Set 1	**Round 1**	**Round 2**	**Round 3**
Squats (page 160)	45 secs on 15 secs rest	45 secs on 15 secs rest	45 secs on 15 secs rest
Dead Bugs (page 182)	45 secs on 15 secs rest	45 secs on 15 secs rest	45 secs on 15 secs rest
Release Press Ups (page 173)	45 secs on 15 secs rest	45 secs on 15 secs rest	45 secs on 15 secs rest
Exercises – Set 2	**Round 1**	**Round 2**	**Round 3**
Lateral Lunges (page 166)	45 secs on 15 secs rest	45 secs on 15 secs rest	45 secs on 15 secs rest
Walkouts (page 184)	45 secs on 15 secs rest	45 secs on 15 secs rest	45 secs on 15 secs rest
Bikes (page 185)	45 secs on 15 secs rest	45 secs on 15 secs rest	45 secs on 15 secs rest

Day 10 Focusing on building core strength in order to protect your lower back and work on the pelvic-floor area.

Abs & Core	Time / Reps / Rounds
Dead Bugs (page 182)	45 secs on / 15 secs rest
Bikes (page 185)	45 secs on / 15 secs rest
Plank Taps (page 183)	45 secs on / 15 secs rest
Bird Dogs (page 197)	45 secs on / 15 secs rest
Twists (page 186)	45 secs on / 15 secs rest
	REPEAT x 3

Loving the plan and healthier new habits are forming!

Charlie

Day 11 Your first lower body workout with weights. Start with the 3kg – if this feels too easy for you, then please use the 5kg. You can use one or both and the workout video will explain this for you clearly.

Lower Body Weights			
Exercises – Set 1	**Round 1**	**Round 2**	**Round 3**
Squats (page 160)	12–14 reps	10–12 reps	8–10 reps
Reverse Lunges (page 162)	8 reps each side	6 reps each side	4 reps each side
Hip Thrusts (page 191)	12–14 reps	10–12 reps	8–10 reps
Exercises – Set 2	**Round 1**	**Round 2**	**Round 3**
Lateral Lunges (page 166)	12–14 reps	10–12 reps	8–10 reps
Sumo Squats (page 170)	12–14 reps	10–12 reps	8–10 reps
Single Leg Thrusts (page 168)	12–14 reps each side	10–12 reps	8–10 reps

Day 12 Using weights you will do a full body workout so you can see how it's possible in 20 minutes to get a great all-over workout with weights for the added extra. To make this sustainable, knowing you can achieve great results with limited time is fundamental.

Full Body Weights			
Exercises – Set 1	**Round 1**	**Round 2**	**Round 3**
Chest Presses (page 187)	12–14 reps	10–12 reps	8–10 reps
Dead Bugs (page 182)	12–14 reps	10–12 reps	8–10 reps
Overhead Presses (page 180)	12–14 reps	10–12 reps	8–10 reps
Exercises – Set 2	**Round 1**	**Round 2**	**Round 3**
Alternating Reverse Lunges Biceps (page 163)	12–14 reps	10–12 reps	8–10 reps
Squat Thrusters (page 180)	12–14 reps	10–12 reps	8–10 reps
Dumbbell RDLs (page 171)	12–14 reps	10–12 reps	8–10 reps

Day 13 A stretching and mobilising day today, giving our body the chance to build and recover from this week's sessions and setting ourselves up for next week.

Stretch & Mobility	Time / Reps / Rounds
Cat Cows (page 197)	x 5
Bird Dogs (page 197)	x 5 each side
Thread the Needles (page 198)	x 5 each side
Hip Flexors (page 199)	45 secs each side x 2
Piriformis Stretches (page 199)	45 secs each side x 2
	REPEAT x 2

Day 14 Finding strength and getting fitter through menopause is about the 360 approach, not just about exercise and diet. Being calm and learning how to control our breath when we are stressed or anxious can play a huge role in managing many of the symptoms of menopause. Day 14 is a wonderful breathwork practice with Anna Gough. Please see video entitled Day 14 via the website or using the QR code on page 97.

DAYS 15–21: LET'S ADD SOME TIME

Over the next 7 days we are going to start making the workouts a little longer and, if you feel able, I would like to encourage you to try to lift heavier weights if you have resisted so far. You will not hurt yourself and the videos will guide you through your form to ensure you are doing it correctly. Also, remember that most of the exercises we will do can be found in Chapter 12 for added reassurance. You will really turn a corner over these next 7 days, so stick with the plan and believe in yourself. You can do this.

DAY 15	DAY 16	DAY 17	DAY 18	DAY 19	DAY 20	DAY 21
UPPER BODY (25 MINS)	BODY-WEIGHT BASICS (20 MINS)	STRETCH & MOBILITY (15 MINS)	UNILAT-ERAL LOWER BODY (25 MINS)	FULL BODY WEIGHTS (25 MINS)	ABS & CORE (15 MINS)	BREATH-WORK MEDIT-ATION

I joined the OYM app recently and love it. I've done weights before but I did the 30-Day Plan as a refresher, and I am on Day 15, feeling stronger already. Loving the meals alongside and I am feeling energised and whole-some. Thank you Kate.

Georgie K

Day 15 We are focusing on adding time to the workouts. You might be able to feel how much stronger you are already and by adding 5 minutes to your sessions, you are testing the body a little more. Remember, this is all about building slowly and leaving a workout with a sense of accomplishment, rather than wishing it had finished sooner.

Upper Body			
Exercises – Set 1	**Round 1**	**Round 2**	**Round 3**
Chest Presses (page 187)	12–14 reps	10–12 reps	8–10 reps
Dead Bugs (page 182)	8 each side	8 each side	8 each side
Tricep Kickbacks (page 179)	12–14 reps	10–12 reps	8–10 reps
Exercises – Set 2	**Round 1**	**Round 2**	**Round 3**
Upright Rows (page 175)	12–14 reps	10–12 reps	8–10 reps
Push Presses (page 188)	12–14 reps	10–12 reps	8–10 reps
Reverse Flys (page 189)	12–14 reps	10–12 reps	8–10 reps

Exercises – Set 3	Round 1	Round 2	Round 3
Plank Taps (page 183)	20 reps (10 each side)	20 reps (10 each side)	20 reps (10 each side)
Twists (page 186)	20 reps (10 each side)	20 reps (10 each side)	20 reps (10 each side)
Mountain Climbers (page 177)	20 reps (10 each side)	20 reps (10 each side)	20 reps (10 each side)

Day 16 This is where you will hopefully feel the big change as we bring it back to a bodyweight session but with added time. You may notice how much easier some of the moves have already become, but we still need to be in control and focus on form however confident we feel.

Bodyweight Basics			
	Round 1	Round 2	Round 3
Squats (page 160)	45 secs on 15 secs rest	45 secs on 15 secs rest	45 secs on 15 secs rest
Release Press Ups (page 173)	45 secs on 15 secs rest	45 secs on 15 secs rest	45 secs on 15 secs rest
Star Steps/Jumps (page 193)	45 secs on 15 secs rest	45 secs on 15 secs rest	45 secs on 15 secs rest
Lunge Jumps (page 164)	45 secs on 15 secs rest	45 secs on 15 secs rest	45 secs on 15 secs rest
Plank Taps (page 183)	45 secs on 15 secs rest	45 secs on 15 secs rest	45 secs on 15 secs rest
Side Shuffles (page 183)	45 secs on 15 secs rest	45 secs on 15 secs rest	45 secs on 15 secs rest

Day 17 A progress day just when you needed it. This is what it is all about – listening to how you feel and ensuring you take the time your body needs to restore. This stretch session will be perfect as you head into your next longer, possibly heavier lower body weighted session.

Stretch & Mobility	Time / Reps / Rounds
Walkouts (page 184)	x 5
Bird Dogs (page 197)	x 5 each side
Thread the Needles (page 198)	x 5 each side
Hip Flexors (page 199)	45 secs each side x 2
Piriformis Stretches (page 199)	45 secs each side x 2
	REPEAT x 2

Day 18 Today we are going to look at unilateral moves because this will help you see how your stronger side (if you have one) often compensates for the weaker one. In working out these imbalances you can help yourself prevent injury and enable your body to be more mobile and flexible, which is key at this stage in life.

Unilateral Training

Have you ever noticed that one side of your body feels stronger? This could be a sign of muscle imbalance. It is not uncommon to have muscular imbalances from carrying out day-to-day activities, such as picking up children and carrying them on one side or a job where you are sitting at home, in the car or at work.

Indicators include uneven balance or flexibility in your body. Poor posture is a cause and symptom of muscle imbalance, which can occur when you sit for long periods or maintain incorrect posture when standing or sitting. Over time, this can leave specific muscles under-worked and weak.

Regular workouts or exercise helps strengthen most muscle groups. The same body parts are sometimes consistently sore after a workout or an activity.

Unilateral training will be beneficial in addressing these imbalances. It is incorporated into the 30-Day Plan because it is an integral part of becoming fitter and stronger and can be a key in injury prevention, too, stopping you from overtraining your dominant side and correcting imbalances.

Treatment for severe muscle imbalance will vary, and if you feel this could be you, please ensure that you seek specific help from a specialist.

Unilateral Lower Body			
Exercises – Set 1	Round 1	Round 2	Round 3
Single Leg Thrusts (page 168)	x 10 each side	x 10 each side	x 10 each side
Reverse Lunges (page 162)	x 6 each side	x 6 each side	x 6 each side
Split Squats (page 162)	x 6 each side	x 6 each side	x 6 each side
Exercises – Set 2	Round 1	Round 2	Round 3
Forward Lunges (page 166)	x 6 each side	x 6 each side	x 6 each side
Single Leg RDLs (page 169)	x 6 each side	x 6 each side	x 6 each side
Lateral Lunges (page 166)	x 6 each side	x 6 each side	x 6 each side

Day 19 Your longest full body weighted workout yet. In adding 5 minutes you will be able to gauge your improvements and feel the gradual progress you are making. Make sure you take notes of how you feel.

Full Body Weights			
Exercises – Set 1	**Round 1**	**Round 2**	**Round 3**
Squats (page 160)	12–14 reps	10–12 reps	8–10 reps
Bent Over Rows (page 174)	12 reps	10 reps	8 reps
Alternating Jackknives (page 187)	x 6 each side	x 6 each side	x 6 each side
Dumbbell Snatches (page 190)	x 6 each side	x 6 each side	x 6 each side
Exercises – Set 2	**Round 1**	**Round 2**	**Round 3**
Push Presses (page 188)	12 reps	10 reps	8 reps
Bear Taps (page 192)	x 10 each side	x 8 each side	x 6 each side
Dumbbell RDLs (page 171)	12 reps	10 reps	8 reps
Mountain Climbers (page 177)	45 secs	45 secs	45 secs

Day 20 Focusing on building core strength in order to protect your lower back and work on the pelvic-floor area

Abs & Core	Time / Reps / Rounds
Dead Bugs (page 182)	45 secs on / 15 secs rest
Bikes (page 185)	45 secs on / 15 secs rest
Plank Taps (page 183)	45 secs on / 15 secs rest
Bird Dogs (page 197)	45 secs on / 15 secs rest
Twists (page 186)	45 secs on / 15 secs rest
	REPEAT x 3

Ready for Day 21. There are so many positives from this plan so far. What has really made a difference is not

eating after 7. My sleep has improved and I feel so much more energised in the morning. I also eliminated processed sugar. I'm feeling an improvement in my tennis elbow, which I've been struggling with for the past 6 months, so happy about this.

Anna G

Day 21 Finding strength and getting fitter through menopause is about the 360 approach, not just about exercise and diet. Being calm and learning how to control our breath when we are stressed or anxious can play a huge role in managing many of the symptoms of menopause. Day 21 is another wonderful breathwork practice with Anna Gough.

DAYS 22-30: LET'S GO HEAVIER AND LONGER

The final few days of the plan. This is where you will be noticing the biggest transformation and be looking ahead at how you can continue with building a fitter, calmer and stronger body, and mind, for life.

You will be encouraged to reach for the heavier weight this week and the classes will be a little bit longer and push you a little more, so you can feel the improvements and see what you are capable of.

It is really fundamental to start thinking this week about how you are going to move forward, and we will talk about this on page 133.

DAY 22	DAY 23	DAY 24	DAY 25	DAY 26	DAY 27	DAY 28
UNILATERAL UPPER BODY (35 MINS)	BODYWEIGHT BASICS (25 MINS)	STRETCH & MOBILITY (15 MINS)	LOWER BODY WEIGHTS (30 MINS)	FULL BODY WEIGHTS (30 MINS)	STRETCH & MOBILITY (15 MINS)	BREATHWORK MEDITATION

DAY 29	DAY 30
ABS & CORE (30 MINS)	FULL BODY WEIGHTS (15 MINS)

Day 22 Unilateral upper body as we haven't done this yet and, just like the lower body session last week, it's important to train this way to help avoid injury and enable the weaker muscles you may have to work harder and not let the stronger ones overcompensate. Each exercise can be done individually or alternating.

Unilateral Upper Body			
Exercises – Set 1	Round 1	Round 2	Round 3
Bent Over Rows (page 174)	10 reps	8 reps	8 reps
Bent Arm Lateral Raises (page 176)	10 reps	8 reps	8 reps
Overhead Presses (page 180)	10 reps	8 reps	8 reps
Exercises – Set 2	Round 1	Round 2	Round 3
Bicep Curls (page 176)	10 reps	8 reps	8 reps
Tricep Kickbacks (page 179)	10 reps	8 reps	8 reps
Front Raises (page 196)	10 reps	8 reps	8 reps

Day 23 This bodyweight session will be greatly appreciated by your upper body after yesterday and will help your recovery process. It will also relieve any aches and pains – motion is lotion remember. It will feel hard but tomorrow we have a stretch session to help.

Bodyweight Basics			
Exercises – Set 1	**Round 1**	**Round 2**	**Round 3**
Squats (page 160)	45 secs on 15 secs rest	45 secs on 15 secs rest	45 secs on 15 secs rest
Frog Pumps (page 167)	45 secs on 15 secs rest	45 secs on 15 secs rest	45 secs on 15 secs rest
Release Press Ups (page 173)	45 secs on 15 secs rest	45 secs on 15 secs rest	45 secs on 15 secs rest
Exercises – Set 2	**Round 1**	**Round 2**	**Round 3**
Lunge Hops (page 164)	45 secs on 15 secs rest	45 secs on 15 secs rest	45 secs on 15 secs rest
Bear Taps (page 192)	45 secs on 15 secs rest	45 secs on 15 secs rest	45 secs on 15 secs rest
Star Steps/Jumps (page 193)	45 secs on 15 secs rest	45 secs on 15 secs rest	45 secs on 15 secs rest
Exercises – Set 3	**Round 1**	**Round 2**	**Round 3**
Mountain Climbers (page 177)	45 secs on 15 secs rest	45 secs on 15 secs rest	45 secs on 15 secs rest
Curtsy Lunges (page 165)	45 secs on 15 secs rest	45 secs on 15 secs rest	45 secs on 15 secs rest
Walkouts/Burpees (page 184)	45 secs on 15 secs rest	45 secs on 15 secs rest	45 secs on 15 secs rest

Day 24 Stretching and mobilising will feel amazing and be fundamental as you are lifting heavier and making changes to your muscles. Seeing how beneficial this feels and using this type of movement on recovery/rest days will help you make progress and stick with your plan.

Stretch & Mobility	Time / Reps / Rounds
Cat Cows (page 197)	x 5
Bird Dogs (page 197)	x 5 each side
Thread the Needles (page 198)	x 5 each side
Hip Flexors (page 199)	45 secs each side x 2
Piriformis Stretches (page 199)	45 secs each side x 2
	REPEAT x 2

Day 25 This final lower body session will combine all the moves we have perfected.

Do you think you can go heavier after these 25 days? Would it be worth investing in heavier weights for when you have finished the plan and you are committed to carrying on this journey?

Lower Body Weights			
Exercises – Set 1	**Round 1**	**Round 2**	**Round 3**
Squats (page 160)	14 reps	12 reps	10 reps
Dumbbell RDLs (page 171)	14 reps	12 reps	10 reps
Curtsy Lunges (page 165)	x 8 each side	x 6 each side	x 4 each side
Exercises – Set 2	**Round 1**	**Round 2**	**Round 3**
Sumo Squats (page 170)	12 reps		
Single Leg Thrusts (page 168)	x 10 each side	x 10 each side	x 10 each side
Lateral Lunges (page 166)	x 6 each side	x 6 each side	x 6 each side

Exercises – Set 3	Round 1	Round 2	Round 3
Kneel Ups (page 194)	x 8 each side	x 6 each side	x 6 each side
Squat Thrusters (page 180)	14 reps	12 reps	10 reps
Dumbbell Swings (page 189)	16 reps	16 reps	16 reps

Day 26 Aiming to use your heavier weights with this full-body workout for 30 minutes will leave you feeling strong and pleased with all the progress you have made. To make this sustainable, know that you can achieve great results with limited time. You will be able to get so much done in these 30 minutes.

Full Body Weights			
Exercises – Set 1	**Round 1**	**Round 2**	**Round 3**
Squats (page 160)	12 reps	10 reps	8 reps
Chest Presses (page 187)	12 reps	10 reps	8 reps
Plank Rotations (page 170)	x 6 each side	x 6 each side	x 6 each side
Exercises – Set 2	**Round 1**	**Round 2**	**Round 3**
Bent Over Rows (page 174)	12 reps	10 reps	8 reps
Curtsy Lunges (page 165)	x 10 each side	x 8 each side	x 6 each side
Lateral Lunges (page 166)	x 6 each side	x 6 each side	x 6 each side
Exercises – Set 3	**Round 1**	**Round 2**	**Round 3**
Upright Rows (page 175)	10 reps	8 reps	6 reps
Squat Thrusters (page 180)	12 reps	10 reps	8 reps
Dumbbell Snatches (page 190)	x 6 each side	x 6 each side	x 6 each side

Day 27 THIS WILL FEEL GOOD. This stretching and mobilising session will feel great as you are lifting heavier. As you head into the final days of this plan, you don't want to be exhausted because it won't be sustainable. Seeing how beneficial this feels and using this type of movement on recovery/rest days will help you make progress and stick with your plan.

Stretch & Mobility	Time / Reps / Rounds
Cat Cows (page 197)	x 5
Bird Dogs (page 197)	x 5 each side
Thread the Needles (page 198)	x 5 each side
Hip Flexors (page 199)	45 secs each side x 2
Piriformis Stretches (page 199)	45 secs each side x 2
	REPEAT x 2

Day 28 Finding strength and getting fitter through menopause is about the 360 approach, not just about exercise and diet. Being calm and learning how to control our breath when we are stressed or anxious can play a huge role in managing many of the symptoms of menopause. Day 28 is a wonderful breathwork practice with Anna Gough.

Day 29 Focusing on building core strength in order to protect your lower back and work on the pelvic-floor area.

Abs & Core	Time / Reps / Rounds
Dead Bugs (page 182)	45 secs on / 15 secs rest
Bikes (page 185)	45 secs on / 15 secs rest
Plank Taps (page 183)	45 secs on / 15 secs rest
Bird Dogs (page 197)	45 secs on / 15 secs rest
Twists (page 186)	45 secs on / 15 secs rest
	REPEAT x 3

Day 30 FINAL DAY – YOU HAVE DONE IT. This will be your hardest full-body cardio weights workout to date, but you will feel a huge sense of accomplishment and hopefully pleasantly surprised at how brilliant it felt.

Full Body Weights			
Exercises – Set 1	**Round 1**	**Round 2**	**Round 3**
Side Shuffles (page 193)	45 secs on 15 secs rest	45 secs on 15 secs rest	45 secs on 15 secs rest
Squat Jumps (page 161)	45 secs on 15 secs rest	45 secs on 15 secs rest	45 secs on 15 secs rest
Mountain Climbers (page 177)	45 secs on 15 secs rest	45 secs on 15 secs rest	45 secs on 15 secs rest
Dead Bugs (page 182)	45 secs on 15 secs rest	45 secs on 15 secs rest	45 secs on 15 secs rest
Exercises – Set 2	**Round 1**	**Round 2**	**Round 3**
Push Presses (page 188)	45 secs on 15 secs rest	45 secs on 15 secs rest	45 secs on 15 secs rest
Reverse Flys (page 189)	45 secs on 15 secs rest	45 secs on 15 secs rest	45 secs on 15 secs rest
Bent Over Rows (page 174)	45 secs on 15 secs rest	45 secs on 15 secs rest	45 secs on 15 secs rest
Exercises – Set 3	**Round 1**	**Round 2**	**Round 3**
Alternating Reverse Lunges (page 162)	45 secs on 15 secs rest	45 secs on 15 secs rest	45 secs on 15 secs rest
Squat Thrusters (page 180)	45 secs on 15 secs rest	45 secs on 15 secs rest	45 secs on 15 secs rest
Dumbbell Swings (page 189)	45 secs on 15 secs rest	45 secs on 15 secs rest	45 secs on 15 secs rest

I'm a 47-year-old single mum to twin boys aged 6, both with ASC, and a full-time teacher. I started finding myself walking around the school grounds breathing to calm myself and feeling very anxious. I put this down to the stress I was under at home due to one of my boys who attends an (amazing) SEN school going through a (very) challenging time. I also had heart palpitations . . . again, I assumed stress from home.

It wasn't until I started working with Kate that I realised it was symptoms of perimenopause and not . . . God love him . . . the extra weight of dealing with my gorgeous boy. I have since started HRT, telling the GP, 'I don't have time to feel like this!' I signed up for Kate's online strength programme and watch religiously all her talks and have just completed sober September and have every intention of carrying on due to the difference it has made.

I had NO idea how challenging menopause could be and the only symptom I knew about was hot flushes.

Still tackling horrifically dry hair but making progress there too!!

Thank you, Kate, for enlightening me and helping me realise this wasn't my 'fault', and certainly not my sons!

Nina F

Progressive overload

When we commit to a new routine, it is essential to try and avoid a plateau. This is where you make good progress at the beginning, but after time your body adapts to the type of exercise you're doing and your progress stops. To avoid this and to ensure we are gradually making progress, overload can be achieved by increasing the frequency, weight and number of repetitions in your lifting sessions. Progressive overload challenges your body and allows you to get stronger. You will get to grips with this and see its role when you start the plan.

While a plateau can be seen as a positive sign that means you've made some gains in your fitness journey, it also signals that it's time to mix things up.

Progressive overload is usually used in strength training, but the same idea can be applied to any type of exercise, including cardiovascular endurance exercises like running.

YOU ARE NOW READY TO CONTINUE THIS JOURNEY TO A FITTER, CALMER, STRONGER YOU

You can move on to the next 30-Day Plan for intermediate to advanced.

This is for those of you who feel you have a good understanding and feel ready to progress.

You could invest in heavier weights or stick with the current ones if you still feel you need time to build more strength.

PLEASE NOTE You could also repeat the beginner's plan if you don't feel ready yet.

CHAPTER 11

The Fitter, Calmer, Stronger in 30 Days Plan for Intermediate/ Advanced

Before you start the intermediate plan, please make sure you have a set of dumbbells ideally ranging anywhere from **5–10kg** as this programme looks at encouraging you to lift heavier weights to ensure you are progressively overloading.

Days 1–7
You may notice a positive change in energy, sleep, confidence, anxiety etc. You are also likely to notice a few aches and pains as you adapt to this new routine and implement a different programme. You will be used to some of the aches and pains you may experience if you already have a good level of fitness and have been exercising regularly.

Days 8–14

You may continue to feel similar benefits as per Days 1–7. Understanding the benefits and putting a new routine into practice is exciting, but remember that even though you may work out regularly, you still want to progress gradually to avoid any injury.

Days 15–28

You will really start to notice and feel how this programme is working and how this could change your life for good. Please keep making notes. The aches and pains may come and go, especially as we introduce longer workouts and potentially increase some of the weights; this is normal and is called DOMS (see page 205). You should now be thinking about how you want to continue and what elements you really want to stick to when it comes to moving forward.

Days 28–30

You will now have made some big changes to your old routine, and you will need to think about what you want to keep and stick to. Have you enjoyed pushing yourself that little bit harder and have you enjoyed the layout of the sessions? Do you need to get heavier weights? Think about all of these so you can plan for the week after you finish the plan.

THE FITTER, STRONGER, CALMER IN 30 DAYS PLAN FOR INTERMEDIATE/ADVANCED

DAY 1	DAY 2	DAY 3	DAY 4	DAY 5	DAY 6	DAY 7
BODY-WEIGHT BASICS (20 MINS)	STRETCH & MOBILITY (15 MINS)	LOWER BODY WEIGHTS (30 MINS)	ABS & CORE (15 MINS)	UPPER BODY WEIGHTS (30 MINS)	STRETCH & MOBILITY (15 MINS)	FULL BODY (30 MINS)

DAY 8	DAY 9	DAY 10	DAY 11	DAY 12	DAY 13	DAY 14
UPPER BODY (40 MINS)	BODY-WEIGHT BASICS (15 MINS)	ABS & CORE (15 MINS)	LOWER BODY (40 MINS)	FULL BODY (40 MINS)	STRETCH & MOBILITY (15 MINS)	BREATH-WORK MEDIT-ATION

DAY 15	DAY 16	DAY 17	DAY 18	DAY 19	DAY 20	DAY 21
UPPER BODY (40 MINS)	BODY-WEIGHT BASICS (20 MINS)	STRETCH & MOBILITY (15 MINS)	UNILAT-ERAL LOWER BODY (40 MINS)	FULL BODY (25 MINS)	ABS & CORE (15 MINS)	BREATH-WORK MEDIT-ATION

DAY 22	DAY 23	DAY 24	DAY 25	DAY 26	DAY 27	DAY 28
UNILAT-ERAL UPPER BODY (35 MINS)	BODY-WEIGHT BASICS (25 MINS)	STRETCH & MOBILITY (15 MINS)	LOWER BODY (35 MINS)	FULL BODY (35 MINS)	ABS & CORE (15 MINS)	BREATH-WORK MEDIT-ATION

DAY 29	DAY 30
FULL BODY WEIGHTED BLAST (20 MINS)	BODY-WEIGHT BASICS (30 MINS)

Warm-up Routine	Time
Walkouts (page 184)	45 secs on / 15 secs rest
Wrist & Ankle Circles	45 secs on / 15 secs rest
Squats (page 160)	45 secs on / 15 secs rest
Release Press Ups (page 173)	45 secs on / 15 secs rest
Plank Rotations (page 170)	45 secs on / 15 secs rest
Star Steps/Jumps (page 193)	45 secs on / 15 secs rest

Cool-down Routine	Time
Piriformis Stretches (page 199)	45 secs on / 15 secs rest
Cat Cows (page 197)	45 secs on / 15 secs rest
Tricep Stretches (page 200)	45 secs on / 15 secs rest
The Baby (page 201)	45 secs on / 15 secs rest
Chest and Bicep Stretches (page 200)	45 secs on / 15 secs rest

Day 1

Bodyweight Basics				
	Round 1	Round 2	Round 3	Round 4
Squats (page 160)	45 secs on 15 secs rest	45 secs on 15 secs rest	45 secs on 15 secs rest	45 secs on 15 secs rest
Dead Bugs (page 182)	45 secs on 15 secs rest	45 secs on 15 secs rest	45 secs on 15 secs rest	45 secs on 15 secs rest
Press Ups (page 172)	45 secs on 15 secs rest	45 secs on 15 secs rest	45 secs on 15 secs rest	45 secs on 15 secs rest
Lateral Lunges (page 166)	45 secs on 15 secs rest	45 secs on 15 secs rest	45 secs on 15 secs rest	45 secs on 15 secs rest
Walkouts (page 184)	45 secs on 15 secs rest	45 secs on 15 secs rest	45 secs on 15 secs rest	45 secs on 15 secs rest

Day 2

Stretch & Mobility	Time / Reps / Rounds
Cat Cows (page 197)	x 5
Bird Dogs (page 197)	x 5 each side
Thread the Needles (page 198)	x 5 each side
Hip Flexors (page 199)	45 secs each side x 2
Piriformis Stretches (page 199)	45 secs each side x 2
	REPEAT x 2

Day 3

Lower Body Weights				
Exercises – Set 1	**Round 1**	**Round 2**	**Round 3**	**Round 4**
Squats (page 160)	12 reps	10 reps	8 reps	6 reps
Reverse Lunges (page 162)	8 reps each side	8 reps each side	6 reps each side	6 reps each side
Hip Thrusts (page 191)	12 reps	10 reps	8 reps	6 reps
Exercises – Set 2	**Round 1**	**Round 2**	**Round 3**	**Round 4**
Good Mornings (page 172)	12 reps	10 reps	8 reps	6 reps
Curtsy Lunges (page 165)	8 reps each side	6 reps each side	6 reps each side	4 reps each side
Split Squats (page 162)	x 10 each side	x 8 each side	x 6 each side	x 4 each side

Day 4

Abs & Core	Time / Reps / Rounds
Dead Bugs (page 182)	45 secs on / 15 secs rest
Bikes (page 185)	45 secs on / 15 secs rest
Plank Taps (page 183)	45 secs on / 15 secs rest
Bird Dogs (page 197)	45 secs on / 15 secs rest
Twists (page 186)	45 secs on / 15 secs rest
	REPEAT x 3

Day 5

Upper Body Weights				
Exercises – Set 1	**Round 1**	**Round 2**	**Round 3**	**Round 4**
Bent Over Rows (page 174)	12 reps	10 reps	8 reps	6 reps
Bent Arm Lateral Raises (page 176)	12 reps	10 reps	8 reps	6 reps
Chest Presses (page 187)	12 reps	10 reps	8 reps	6 reps
Exercises – Set 2	**Round 1**	**Round 2**	**Round 3**	**Round 4**
Bicep Curls (page 176)	12 reps	10 reps	8 reps	6 reps
Tricep Kickbacks (page 179)	12 reps	10 reps	8 reps	6 reps
Overhead Presses (page 180)	12 reps	10 reps	8 reps	6 reps

Day 6

Stretch & Mobility	Time / Reps / Rounds
Cat Cows (page 197)	x 5
Bird Dogs (page 197)	x 5 each side
Thread the Needles (page 198)	x 5 each side
Hip Flexors (page 199)	45 secs each side x 2
Piriformis Stretches (page 199)	45 secs each side x 2
	REPEAT x 2

Day 7

Full Body			
Exercises – Set 1	**Round 1**	**Round 2**	**Round 3**
Side Shuffles (page 193)	45 secs on 15 secs rest	45 secs on 15 secs rest	45 secs on 15 secs rest
Squat Jumps (page 161)	45 secs on 15 secs rest	45 secs on 15 secs rest	45 secs on 15 secs rest
Mountain Climbers (page 177)	45 secs on 15 secs rest	45 secs on 15 secs rest	45 secs on 15 secs rest
Dead Bugs (page 182)	45 secs on 15 secs rest	45 secs on 15 secs rest	45 secs on 15 secs rest
Exercises – Set 2	**Round 1**	**Round 2**	**Round 3**
Push Presses (page 188)	45 secs on 15 secs rest	45 secs on 15 secs rest	45 secs on 15 secs rest
Reverse Flys (page 189)	45 secs on 15 secs rest	45 secs on 15 secs rest	45 secs on 15 secs rest
Bent Over Rows (page 174)	45 secs on 15 secs rest	45 secs on 15 secs rest	45 secs on 15 secs rest
Exercises – Set 3	**Round 1**	**Round 2**	**Round 3**
Alternating Reverse Lunges (page 162)	45 secs on 15 secs rest	45 secs on 15 secs rest	45 secs on 15 secs rest
Squat Thrusters (page 180)	45 secs on 15 secs rest	45 secs on 15 secs rest	45 secs on 15 secs rest
Dumbbell Swings (page 189)	45 secs on 15 secs rest	45 secs on 15 secs rest	45 secs on 15 secs rest

DAYS 8-14

DAY 8	DAY 9	DAY 10	DAY 11	DAY 12	DAY 13	DAY 14
UPPER BODY (40 MINS)	BODY-WEIGHT BASICS (15 MINS)	ABS & CORE (15 MINS)	LOWER BODY (40 MINS)	FULL BODY (40 MINS)	STRETCH & MOBILITY (15 MINS)	BREATH-WORK MEDIT-ATION

Day 8

Upper Body				
Exercises – Set 1	**Round 1**	**Round 2**	**Round 3**	**Round 4**
Chest Presses (page 187)	14 reps	12 reps	10 reps	8 reps
Dead Bugs (page 182)	10 reps (5 each side)	10 reps (5 each side)	10 reps (5 each side)	10 reps (5 each side)
Tricep Kickbacks (page 179)	12 reps	10 reps	8 reps	6 reps
Exercises – Set 2	**Round 1**	**Round 2**	**Round 3**	**Round 4**
Upright Rows (page 175)	14 reps	12 reps	10 reps	8 reps
Push Presses (page 188)	14 reps	12 reps	10 reps	8 reps
Reverse Flys (page 189)	14 reps	12 reps	10 reps	8 reps
Exercises – Set 3	**Round 1**	**Round 2**	**Round 3**	**Round 4**
Plank Taps (page 183)	20 reps (10 each side)	20 reps (10 each side)	20 reps (10 each side)	20 reps (10 each side)
Twists (page 186)	10 reps (5 each side)	10 reps (5 each side)	10 reps (5 each side)	10 reps (5 each side)
Slow Mountain Climbers (page 177)	20 reps (10 each side)	20 reps (10 each side)	20 reps (10 each side)	20 reps (10 each side)

Day 9

Bodyweight Basics			
Exercises	Round 1	Round 2	Round 3
Alternating Reverse Lunges Overhead (page 164)	45 secs on 15 secs rest	45 secs on 15 secs rest	45 secs on 15 secs rest
Squat Pulses (page 161)	45 secs on 15 secs rest	45 secs on 15 secs rest	45 secs on 15 secs rest
Single Leg Thrusts (switch legs half way) (page 168)	45 secs on 15 secs rest	45 secs on 15 secs rest	45 secs on 15 secs rest
Frog Pumps (page 167)	45 secs on 15 secs rest	45 secs on 15 secs rest	45 secs on 15 secs rest
Curtsy Lunges (page 165)	45 secs on 15 secs rest	45 secs on 15 secs rest	45 secs on 15 secs rest

Day 10

Abs & Core	Time / Reps / Rounds
Dead Bugs (page 182)	45 secs on / 15 secs rest
Bikes (page 185)	45 secs on / 15 secs rest
Plank Taps (page 183)	45 secs on / 15 secs rest
Bird Dogs (page 197)	45 secs on / 15 secs rest
Twists (page 186)	45 secs on / 15 secs rest
	REPEAT x 3

Day 11

Lower Body				
Exercises – Set 1	**Round 1**	**Round 2**	**Round 3**	**Round 4**
Squats (page 160)	14 reps	12 reps	10 reps	8 reps
Single Leg RDLs (page 169)	8 reps each side	8 reps each side	6 reps each side	6 reps each side
Curtsy Lunges (page 165)	12 reps (6 each side)	12 reps (6 each side)	12 reps (6 each side)	12 reps (6 each side)
Exercises – Set 2	**Round 1**	**Round 2**	**Round 3**	**Round 4**
Sumo Squats (page 170)	14 reps	12 reps	10 reps	8 reps
Single Leg Thrusts (page 168)	20 reps (10 each side)	20 reps (10 each side)	20 reps (10 each side)	20 reps (10 each side)
Lateral Lunges (page 166)	16 reps (8 each side)	16 reps (8 each side)	12 reps (6 each side)	12 reps (6 each side)
Exercises – Set 3	**Round 1**	**Round 2**	**Round 3**	**Round 4**
Kneel Ups (page 194)	16 reps (8 each side)	16 reps (8 each side)	12 reps (6 each side)	12 reps (6 each side)
Squat Thrusters (page 180)	14 reps	12 reps	10 reps	8 reps
Dumbbell Swings (page 189)	16 reps	16 reps	14 reps	12 reps

Day 12

Full Body			
Exercises – Set 1	**Round 1**	**Round 2**	**Round 3**
Side Shuffles (page 193)	45 secs on 15 secs rest	45 secs on 15 secs rest	45 secs on 15 secs rest
Squat Jumps (page 161)	45 secs on 15 secs rest	45 secs on 15 secs rest	45 secs on 15 secs rest
Mountain Climbers (page 177)	45 secs on 15 secs rest	45 secs on 15 secs rest	45 secs on 15 secs rest
Dead Bugs (page 182)	45 secs on 15 secs rest	45 secs on 15 secs rest	45 secs on 15 secs rest
Exercises – Set 2	**Round 1**	**Round 2**	**Round 3**
Push Presses (page 188)	45 secs on 15 secs rest	45 secs on 15 secs rest	45 secs on 15 secs rest
Reverse Flys (page 189)	45 secs on 15 secs rest	45 secs on 15 secs rest	45 secs on 15 secs rest
Bent Over Rows (page 174)	45 secs on 15 secs rest	45 secs on 15 secs rest	45 secs on 15 secs rest
Exercises – Set 3	**Round 1**	**Round 2**	**Round 3**
Alternating Reverse Lunges (page 162)	45 secs on 15 secs rest	45 secs on 15 secs rest	45 secs on 15 secs rest
Squat Thrusters (page 180)	45 secs on 15 secs rest	45 secs on 15 secs rest	45 secs on 15 secs rest
Dumbbell Swings (page 189)	45 secs on 15 secs rest	45 secs on 15 secs rest	45 secs on 15 secs rest

Day 13

Stretch & Mobility	Time / Reps / Rounds
Cat Cow (page 197)	x 5
Bird Dogs (page 197)	x 5 each side
Thread the Needles (page 198)	x 5 each side
Hip Flexors (page 199)	45 secs each side x 2
Piriformis Stretches (page 199)	45 secs each side x 2
	REPEAT x 2

Day 14 Finding strength and getting fitter through menopause is about the 360 approach, not just about exercise and diet. Being calm and learning how to control our breath when we are stressed or anxious can play a huge role in managing many of the symptoms of menopause, as well as helping with our overall well-being, which in turn can help you stay committed to a workout. Day 14 is another wonderful breathwork practice with Anna Gough.

DAYS 15–21

DAY 15	DAY 16	DAY 17	DAY 18	DAY 19	DAY 20	DAY 21
UPPER BODY (40 MINS)	BODY-WEIGHT BASICS (20 MINS)	STRETCH & MOBILITY (15 MINS)	UNILAT-ERAL LOWER BODY (40 MINS)	FULL BODY (25 MINS)	ABS & CORE (15 MINS)	BREATH-WORK MEDIT-ATION

Day 15

Upper Body Workout				
Exercises – Set 1	**Round 1**	**Round 2**	**Round 3**	**Round 4**
Chest Presses (page 187)	14 reps	12 reps	10 reps	8 reps
Dead Bugs (page 182)	12 reps (6 each side)	12 reps (6 each side)	12 reps (6 each side)	12 reps (6 each side)
Tricep Kickbacks (page 179)	12 reps	10 reps	8 reps	6 reps
Exercises – Set 2	**Round 1**	**Round 2**	**Round 3**	**Round 4**
Upright Rows (page 175)	14 reps	12 reps	10 reps	8 reps
Push Presses (page 188)	14 reps	12 reps	10 reps	8 reps
Reverse Flys (page 189)	14 reps	12 reps	10 reps	8 reps
Exercises – Set 3	**Round 1**	**Round 2**	**Round 3**	**Round 4**
Plank Taps (page 183)	12 reps (6 each side)	12 reps (6 each side)	12 reps (6 each side)	12 reps (6 each side)
Twists (page 186)	20 reps (10 each side)	20 reps (10 each side)	20 reps (10 each side)	20 reps (10 each side)

Slow Mountain Climbers (page 177)	20 reps (10 each side)	20 reps (10 each side)	20 reps (10 each side)	20 reps (10 each side)

Day 16

Body-weight Basics				
Exercises	**Round 1**	**Round 2**	**Round 3**	**Round 4**
Squats (page 160)	45 secs on 15 secs rest	45 secs on 15 secs rest	45 secs on 15 secs rest	45 secs on 15 secs rest
Release Press Ups (page 173)	45 secs on 15 secs rest	45 secs on 15 secs rest	45 secs on 15 secs rest	45 secs on 15 secs rest
Star Steps/ Jumps (page 193)	45 secs on 15 secs rest	45 secs on 15 secs rest	45 secs on 15 secs rest	45 secs on 15 secs rest
Lunge Jumps (page 164)	45 secs on 15 secs rest	45 secs on 15 secs rest	45 secs on 15 secs rest	45 secs on 15 secs rest
Plank Taps (page 183)	45 secs on 15 secs rest	45 secs on 15 secs rest	45 secs on 15 secs rest	45 secs on 15 secs rest
Side Shuffles (page 193)	45 secs on 15 secs rest	45 secs on 15 secs rest	45 secs on 15 secs rest	45 secs on 15 secs rest

Day 17

Stretch & Mobility	**Time / Reps / Rounds**
Walkouts (page 184)	x 5
Bird Dogs (page 197)	x 5 each side
Thread the Needles (page 198)	x 5 each side
Hip Flexors (page 199)	45 secs each side x 2
Piriformis Stretches (page 199)	45 secs each side x 2
	REPEAT x 2

Day 18 Today we are going to look at unilateral moves (see page 122) because this will help you see how your stronger side (if you have one) often compensates for your weaker one. In working out these imbalances you can help prevent injury and enable your body to be more mobile and flexible, which is key at this stage in life.

Exercises – Set 1	Round 1	Round 2	Round 3	Round 4
Single Leg Thrusts (page 168)	20 reps (10 each side)	20 reps (10 each side)	20 reps (10 each side)	20 reps (10 each side)
Reverse Lunges (page 162)	2 reps (6 each side)	2 reps (6 each side)	12 reps (6 each side)	12 reps (6 each side)
Split Squats (page 162)	12 reps (6 each side)	12 reps (6 each side)	12 reps (6 each side)	12 reps (6 each side)
Exercises – Set 2	Round 1	Round 2	Round 3	Round 4
Forward Lunges (page 166)	12 reps (6 each side)	12 reps (6 each side)	12 reps (6 each side)	12 reps (6 each side)
Single Leg RDLs (page 169)	12 reps (6 each side)	12 reps (6 each side)	12 reps (6 each side)	12 reps (6 each side)
Lateral Lunges (page 166)	12 reps (6 each side)	12 reps (6 each side)	12 reps (6 each side)	12 reps (6 each side)
Plank Taps (page 183)	20 reps (10 each side)	20 reps (10 each side)	20 reps (10 each side)	20 reps (10 each side)

Day 19

Full Body			
Exercises – Set 1	**Round 1**	**Round 2**	**Round 3**
Squats (page 160)	45 secs on 15 secs rest	45 secs on 15 secs rest	45 secs on 15 secs rest
Bent Over Rows (page 174)	45 secs on 15 secs rest	45 secs on 15 secs rest	45 secs on 15 secs rest
Alternating Jackknives (page 187)	45 secs on 15 secs rest	45 secs on 15 secs rest	45 secs on 15 secs rest
Dumbbell Snatches (page 190)	45 secs on 15 secs rest	45 secs on 15 secs rest	45 secs on 15 secs rest
Exercises – Set 2	**Round 1**	**Round 2**	**Round 3**
Push Presses (page 188)	45 secs on 15 secs rest	45 secs on 15 secs rest	45 secs on 15 secs rest
Bear Taps (page 192)	45 secs on 15 secs rest	45 secs on 15 secs rest	45 secs on 15 secs rest
Single Leg RDLs, switching sides halfway (page 169)	45 secs on 15 secs rest	45 secs on 15 secs rest	45 secs on 15 secs rest
Upright Rows (page 175)	45 secs on 15 secs rest	45 secs on 15 secs rest	45 secs on 15 secs rest
Mountain Climbers (page 177)	45 secs on 15 secs rest	45 secs on 15 secs rest	45 secs on 15 secs rest

Day 20

Abs & Core	Time / Reps / Rounds
Dead Bugs (page 182)	45 secs on / 15 secs rest
Bikes (page 185)	45 secs on / 15 secs rest
Plank Taps (page 183)	45 secs on / 15 secs rest
Bird Dogs (page 197)	45 secs on / 15 secs rest
Twists (page 186)	45 secs on / 15 secs rest
	REPEAT x 3

Day 21 Finding strength and getting fitter through menopause is about the 360 approach, not just about exercise and diet. Being calm and learning how to control our breath when we are stressed or anxious can play a huge role in managing many of the symptoms of menopause, as well as helping with our overall well-being, which in turn can help you stay committed to a workout. Day 21 is another wonderful breathwork practice with Anna Gough.

DAYS 22–30

DAY 22	DAY 23	DAY 24	DAY 25	DAY 26	DAY 27	DAY 28
UNILAT-ERAL UPPER BODY (35 MINS)	BODY-WEIGHT BASICS (25 MINS)	STRETCH & MOBILITY (15 MINS)	LOWER BODY (35 MINS)	FULL BODY WEIGHTS (35 MINS)	ABS & CORE (15 MINS)	BREATH-WORK MEDIT-ATION

DAY 29	DAY 30
BODY-WEIGHT BASICS (25 MINS)	FULL BODY BLAST (BODY-WEIGHT) (30 MINS)

Day 22

Unilateral Upper Body			
Exercises – Set 1	Round 1	Round 2	Round 3
Bent Over Rows, individually (page 174)	12 reps each side	10 reps each side	8 reps each side
Bent Arm Lateral Raises, individually (page 176)	12 reps each side	10 reps each side	8 reps each side
Overhead Presses, individually (page 180)	12 reps each side	10 reps each side	8 reps each side
Exercises – Set 2	Round 1	Round 2	Round 3
Bicep Curls (page 176)	12 reps each side	10 reps each side	8 reps each side
Tricep Kickbacks (page 179)	12 reps each side	10 reps each side	8 reps each side
Alternating Front Raises (page 196)	12 reps each side	10 reps each side	8 reps each side

Unilateral upper body as we haven't done this yet and, just like the lower body session last week, it's important to train this way to help avoid injury and enable the weaker muscles you may have to work harder and not let the stronger ones overcompensate.

Day 23

Bodyweight Basics			
Exercises – Set 1	**Round 1**	**Round 2**	**Round 3**
Squats (page 160)	45 secs on 15 secs rest	45 secs on 15 secs rest	45 secs on 15 secs rest
Frog Pumps (page 167)	45 secs on 15 secs rest	45 secs on 15 secs rest	45 secs on 15 secs rest
Release Press Ups (page 173)	45 secs on 15 secs rest	45 secs on 15 secs rest	45 secs on 15 secs rest
Exercises – Set 2	**Round 1**	**Round 2**	**Round 3**
Lunge Hops (page 164)	45 secs on 15 secs rest	45 secs on 15 secs rest	45 secs on 15 secs rest
Bear Taps (page 192)	45 secs on 15 secs rest	45 secs on 15 secs rest	45 secs on 15 secs rest
Star Steps/Jumps (page 193)	45 secs on 15 secs rest	45 secs on 15 secs rest	45 secs on 15 secs rest
Exercises – Set 3	**Round 1**	**Round 2**	**Round 3**
Mountain Climbers (page 177)	45 secs on 15 secs rest	45 secs on 15 secs rest	45 secs on 15 secs rest
Curtsy Lunges (page 165)	45 secs on 15 secs rest	45 secs on 15 secs rest	45 secs on 15 secs rest
Walkouts/Burpees (page 184)	45 secs on 15 secs rest	45 secs on 15 secs rest	45 secs on 15 secs rest

Day 24

Stretch & Mobility	Time / Reps / Rounds
Cat Cows (page 197)	x 5
Bird Dogs (page 197)	x 5 each side
Thread the Needles (page 198)	x 5 each side
Hip Flexors (page 199)	45 secs each side x 2
Piriformis Stretches (page 199)	45 secs each side x 2
	REPEAT x 2

Day 25

Lower Body			
Exercises – Set 1	**Round 1**	**Round 2**	**Round 3**
Squats (page 160)	12 reps	10 reps	8 reps
Dumbbell RDLs (page 171)	12 reps	10 reps	8 reps
Curtsy Lunges (page 165)	16 reps (8 each side)	12 reps (6 each side)	12 reps (6 each side)
Frog Pumps (page 167)	30 pumps	30 pumps	30 pumps
Exercises – Set 2	**Round 1**	**Round 2**	**Round 3**
Sumo Squats (page 170)	12 reps	10 reps	8 reps
Single Leg Thrusts (page 168)	20 reps (10 each side)	20 reps (10 each side)	20 reps (10 each side)
Lateral Lunges (page 166)	12 reps (6 each side)	12 reps (6 each side)	12 reps (6 each side)
Exercises – Set 3	**Round 1**	**Round 2**	**Round 3**
Kneel Ups (page 194)	12 reps (6 each side)	10 reps (5 each side)	8 reps (4 each side)
Squat Thrusters (page 180)	10 reps	8 reps	6 reps
Dumbbell Swings (page 189)	16 reps	16 reps	16 reps

Day 26

Full Body			
Exercises – Set 1	**Round 1**	**Round 2**	**Round 3**
Squats (page 160)	45 secs on 15 secs rest	45 secs on 15 secs rest	45 secs on 15 secs rest
Chest Presses (page 187)	45 secs on 15 secs rest	45 secs on 15 secs rest	45 secs on 15 secs rest
Plank Rotations (page 170)	45 secs on 15 secs rest	45 secs on 15 secs rest	45 secs on 15 secs rest
Exercises – Set 2	**Round 1**	**Round 2**	**Round 3**
Bent Over Rows (page 174)	45 secs on 15 secs rest	45 secs on 15 secs rest	45 secs on 15 secs rest
Curtsy Lunges (page 165)	45 secs on 15 secs rest	45 secs on 15 secs rest	45 secs on 15 secs rest
Lateral Lunges (page 166)	45 secs on 15 secs rest	45 secs on 15 secs rest	45 secs on 15 secs rest
Exercises – Set 3	**Round 1**	**Round 2**	**Round 3**
Upright Rows (page 175)	45 secs on 15 secs rest	45 secs on 15 secs rest	45 secs on 15 secs rest
Squat Thrusters (page 180)	45 secs on 15 secs rest	45 secs on 15 secs rest	45 secs on 15 secs rest
Dumbbell Snatches (page 190)	45 secs on 15 secs rest (switch half way)	45 secs on 15 secs rest (switch half way)	45 secs on 15 secs rest (switch half way)

Day 27

Abs & Core	Time / Reps / Rounds
Dead Bugs (page 182)	45 secs on / 15 secs rest
Bikes (page 185)	45 secs on / 15 secs rest
Plank Taps (page 183)	45 secs on / 15 secs rest
Bird Dogs (page 197)	45 secs on / 15 secs rest
Twists (page 186)	45 secs on / 15 secs rest
	REPEAT x 3

Day 28 Finding strength and getting fitter through menopause is about the 360 approach, not just about exercise and diet. Being calm and learning how to control our breath when we are stressed or anxious can play a huge role in managing many of the symptoms of menopause, as well as helping with our overall well-being, which in turn can help you stay committed to a workout. Day 28 is another wonderful breathwork practice with Anna Gough.

Day 29

Full Body Blast Weights			
Exercises – Set 1	**Round 1**	**Round 2**	**Round 3**
Side Shuffles (page 193)	45 secs on 15 secs rest	45 secs on 15 secs rest	45 secs on 15 secs rest
Squat Jumps (page 161)	45 secs on 15 secs rest	45 secs on 15 secs rest	45 secs on 15 secs rest
Mountain Climbers (page 177)	45 secs on 15 secs rest	45 secs on 15 secs rest	45 secs on 15 secs rest
Dead Bugs (page 182)	45 secs on 15 secs rest	45 secs on 15 secs rest	45 secs on 15 secs rest
Exercises – Set 2	**Round 1**	**Round 2**	**Round 3**
Push Presses (page 188)	45 secs on 15 secs rest	45 secs on 15 secs rest	45 secs on 15 secs rest

Reverse Flys (page 189)	45 secs on 15 secs rest	45 secs on 15 secs rest	45 secs on 15 secs rest
Bent Over Rows (page 184)	45 secs on 15 secs rest	45 secs on 15 secs rest	45 secs on 15 secs rest
Exercises – Set 3	**Round 1**	**Round 2**	**Round 3**
Alternating Reverse Lunges (page 162)	45 secs on 15 secs rest	45 secs on 15 secs rest	45 secs on 15 secs rest
Squat Thrusters (page 180)	45 secs on 15 secs rest	45 secs on 15 secs rest	45 secs on 15 secs rest
Dumbbell Swings (page 189)	45 secs on 15 secs rest	45 secs on 15 secs rest	45 secs on 15 secs rest

Day 30

Body-weight Basics				
Exercises	**Round 1**	**Round 2**	**Round 3**	**Round 4**
Squats (page 160)	45 secs on 15 secs rest	45 secs on 15 secs rest	45 secs on 15 secs rest	45 secs on 15 secs rest
Release Press Ups (page 173)	45 secs on 15 secs rest	45 secs on 15 secs rest	45 secs on 15 secs rest	45 secs on 15 secs rest
Star Steps/ Jumps (page 193)	45 secs on 15 secs rest	45 secs on 15 secs rest	45 secs on 15 secs rest	45 secs on 15 secs rest
Lunge Jumps (page 164)	45 secs on 15 secs rest	45 secs on 15 secs rest	45 secs on 15 secs rest	45 secs on 15 secs rest
Plank Taps (page 183)	45 secs on 15 secs rest	45 secs on 15 secs rest	45 secs on 15 secs rest	45 secs on 15 secs rest
Side Shuffles (page 193)	45 secs on 15 secs rest	45 secs on 15 secs rest	45 secs on 15 secs rest	45 secs on 15 secs rest

CHAPTER 12

The Exercises

These are all the exercises that we will be using in the plan. I have given you detailed explanations of how to execute them and the illustrations will be helpful.

However, I would love to encourage you to follow the workouts in real time with the videos as you will then see me doing the exercises, which can often be more helpful.

How to avoid injuries

One of your biggest concerns when starting a new programme should be avoiding injuries, so finding your form when executing some of the most common moves included in the plan is important. You may experience imbalances that prevent you from completing your full range of movement, and we will try to address these by looking at technique.

If you find some moves particularly challenging, it would be worth seeking advice from a physiotherapist on correcting your technique to avoid injury and progress better. Taking the time and energy to do this now can save you from long-term injuries. Make sure you look at the diagrams and if you can, use the follow-along videos for extra guidance on form and technique.

It's important to know that more complicated moves don't necessarily mean better progress. Instead, focus on building balance, mobility and strength by using the functional patterns of movement as discussed earlier in the book (see Chapter 8). And it's also crucial to understand that achieving perfect technique takes time and effort.

Your core and why do we always talk about it?

We hear the term 'core' all the time when it comes to exercise. But what does that term mean?

Your core is not just your stomach muscles. Your core is made up of many different muscles and includes your pelvis, lower back, hips and stomach. It is essentially the central part of your body. When we work this part of our body, we create better balance, mobility and stability. The core muscles provide support and strength for your abdomen and hold you upright.[30]

To ensure you are 'engaging' your core properly in a workout, it is crucial to engage both your stomach and back muscles simultaneously. Any exercise that achieves this is classified as a core exercise, such as using free weights while maintaining a stable core. This not only trains and strengthens multiple muscles but also your core muscles.

You may experience lower back pain or feel like you have bad balance when executing some exercises. This

can be down to not having a strong core, which is a
fundamental component of building mobility and stability
and why we will work on it throughout the 30-Day Plan.
If you experience sudden or continuous pain please seek
help from your GP.

Compound Movements

Compound movements engage all of the main muscle groups in
your body, meaning you are using more than one muscle group at
a time. Compound exercises are a great place to start if you have
relatively general goals like improving your overall cardiovascular
fitness and increasing your strength.

A squat, for example, uses your core, quads, hamstrings, glutes
and hip flexors.

Squats

It's hard not to notice how perfectly toddlers squat. That's because
squatting is a fundamental movement pattern that requires multiple joint and muscle integration. As we age, we tend to forget this
movement in favour of bending over.

However, incorporating squats into your exercise routine can
lead to numerous benefits. Not only can squats improve your
overall exercise performance, but they can also reduce your risk
of injury and help you move more efficiently throughout the day.

Additionally, many of the muscles used in squats are essential
for everyday activities, such as walking, climbing stairs and carrying heavy loads.

How to do it: To begin, position your feet at shoulder width
and let your arms rest at your sides. As you maintain a strong
core and upright posture with your neck in a neutral position,
slowly lower your body by bending your knees and pushing

your hips backwards. Pause once your thighs are parallel to the ground before standing back up and squeezing your glutes. This movement can be made more challenging by adding weight.

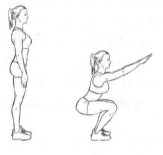

What are we working? Bum (Glutes), Legs, Core

Squat Jumps

As above but power yourself up through your heels and come off the ground in an explosive movement. Land back softly into the squat position, bending gently through the knees and then another explosive movement back up again. Do the desired reps.

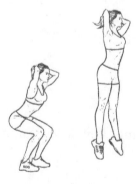

Squat Pulses

Same technique as squats but hold the squat at the bottom and gently pulse up and down without coming all the way up.

Reverse Lunges

Incorporating reverse lunges into your exercise routine can have numerous benefits. Not only do they activate your core, glutes and hamstrings, but they also put less stress on your joints. Additionally, reverse lunges provide more stability in your front legs, making them an excellent option for individuals with knee concerns, difficulty balancing or less hip mobility. By switching up the direction of your movement and training your muscles to work differently, reverse lunges can help improve your balance and overall fitness.

How to do it: Stand up straight with your feet shoulder-width apart and hold a pair of dumbbells or kettlebells at your sides. Take a step backwards with your left leg and lunge as far as you comfortably can while dropping your hips downward. When you reach the bottom of the lunge, push back to the starting position with both legs at the same time. Repeat the lunge with your right leg and alternate legs for the desired number of repetitions. Remember to maintain proper form and breath control throughout the exercise.

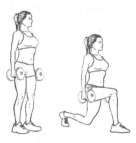

What are we working? Bum (Glutes), Legs, Core

Split Squats

The split squat looks very similar to a lunge. However, the feet stay in one place for the most part during this exercise.

How to do it: Set up in a split stance position while gripping dumbbells by your side with a neutral grip. Descend by flexing both knees simultaneously and continue until the back knee touches the ground directly beneath the hip. Drive through the front foot and extend the knee as you return to the starting position. Repeat on other side.

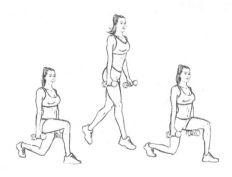

What are we working? Bum (Glutes), Legs, Core

Reverse Lunges Biceps
Same technique as reverse lunges but adding a bicep curl for the extra challenge. As you step into the reverse lunge, lift the arms into a bicep curl.

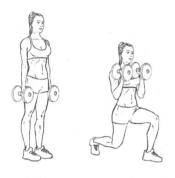

Reverse Lunges Overhead
Same technique as reverse lunges but lift the dumbbells overhead as you come up and, using your momentum, push through the knee at the same time.

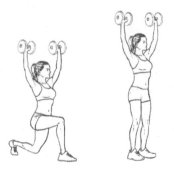

Lunge Jumps
Take a large step backward and lower your hips, so that your back knee is just above the floor and your front thigh is parallel to the floor. Jump into the air and switch leg positions. Jump again and return to the starting position.

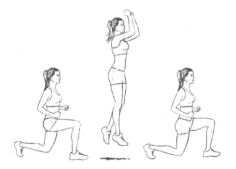

Lunge Hops
Similar to lunge jumps, lunge hops work the same group of muscles but unilaterally.

How to do it: While standing, lunge back with one leg, by stepping back and bending your front leg. Once your back knee is close to the ground, explode up by pressing the front foot through the floor and hopping up as you drive your back knee up into the air. Repeat on the other side.

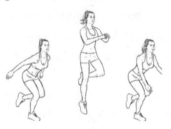

Curtsy Lunges

The curtsy lunge is great for building lower body strength and stability. The gluteus medius (GM) is an important muscle for stability but isn't directly targeted in squats and lunges.

How to do it: Stand with your feet shoulder-width apart and your arms down at your sides. Putting your weight into your right foot, step back and around with your left foot – almost as if you're curtsying – allowing your arms to come up in front of you to a comfortable position. To make sure you are balanced, make sure you have room between your front heel and bent knee. Stop lunging when your right thigh is parallel to the ground. Begin to straighten your right leg, pushing up through your heel, and returning your left foot to the starting position.

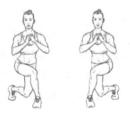

What are we working? Bum (Glutes), Legs, Core, Hip adductors

Lateral Lunges

One exercise that can help strengthen and improve mobility is the lateral or side-stepping lunge. Unlike traditional lunges that move forward or backwards, this exercise involves stepping to the side. This unilateral movement is important because many of our daily activities involve only forward or backward movements. Including lateral work in your routine ensures our bodies are strong and healthy enough to move in every direction to help with balance and stability.

How to do it: Stand with your feet hip-width apart. Take a big step to the side with your left leg, then bend your right knee, push your hips back and lower until your right knee is bent 90 degrees. This should take around 2 seconds. Push back to the starting position. Alternate sides and add weight for more strength gains.

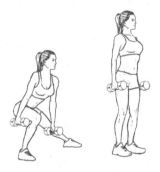

What are we working? Hamstrings, Quads, Inner thigh muscles (adductors), Outer glutes

Forward Lunges

The forward lunge works your hamstrings, quadriceps, hip flexor muscles, gluteus maximus, and the muscles in your inner thighs. They can help increase your stability in your core and back and are a great way to focus on balance.

How to do it: Stand tall with feet hip-width apart. Engage your core. Take a big step forward with your right leg. Lower your body until the right thigh is parallel to the floor and the right shin is vertical. Press into the right heel to drive back up to the starting position.

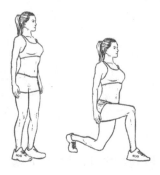

What are we working? Hamstrings, Quads, Inner thigh muscles (adductors), Outer glutes

Frog Pumps

The frog pump is a beneficial glute exercise. The aim of the frog pump exercise is to isolate and strengthen your glute muscles. It engages your gluteus maximus (the largest butt muscle, which functions to extend your hips and rotate your legs outward) and gluteus minimus (the smallest butt muscle, which lies beneath the gluteus maximus and gluteus medius) and allows you to move your legs outward and rotate them inward, offering good mobility.

How to do it: Lie on your back and bring the soles of your feet together into a 'frog' position, scooting your feet as close to your bum as possible. If doing the exercise with just body weight, make fists with your hands and keep elbows on the floor so your fore-arms are perpendicular to the ground. If using a dumbbell, hold it on either end while resting it on the hips. Draw your belly button down towards the floor to engage the midsection and press your lower back into the floor.

Then, keeping your chin tucked into your neck, ribs down and shoulders on the ground, press down into the floor with the edges of your feet and squeeze the glutes to thrust your hips towards the ceiling. Pause at the top before lowering your butt back down to the floor with control.

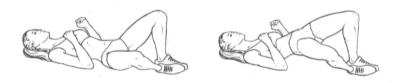

What are we working? Bum (Glutes), Legs, Core

Single Leg Thrusts

The single leg hip thrust is a great unilateral exercise for targeting the glutes. Working each side separately allows you to isolate your glutes, which can be beneficial. This exercise has a low risk of injury and is great for all fitness levels.

How to do it: Start by lying on your back with one knee bent at about 90 degrees and the foot of the same leg flat on the floor – this will be your working leg. Lift your other leg, bending your knee until both your hip and knee form a 90-degree angle. Lay your arms out flat on the floor. Focus on using your upper back as a pivot. Contract the glute of the working leg and lift your hips until they're in line with your torso. Briefly hold this position while continuing to squeeze your glute, and finally, return to the starting position.

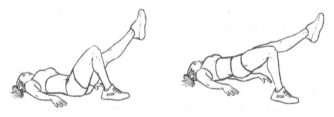

What are we working? Glutes, but also supporting muscles including Hamstrings, Quads, Adductors

Single Leg RDLs (Romanian Deadlifts)

The single leg RDL helps to eliminate strength imbalances on the left and right sides of the body and improves lower-body stability, which may protect the knees from injury. It is one of the best all-around exercises for developing lower-body strength and improving long-term health.

How to do it: Stand balancing on your left leg and hold your dumbbells with palms facing your thighs. Hinge your hips back as if you were pushing a cupboard closed with your bottom and allow your left knee to bend slightly. Your right leg should be straight (it's OK if there's a slight bend in the knee) and in line with your body throughout the rep. Keeping your back flat and squeezing the shoulder blades together to keep a neutral spine, continue to bend at the waist until the dumbbell is at about mid-shin height. Drive through your heel and push your hips forward to stand up to the starting position. This exercise can be executed with one dumbbell, or with one in each hand.

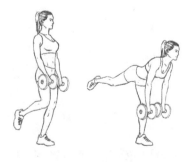

What are we working? Glutes, Hamstrings, Lower back

Sumo Squats

A squat is an excellent move for boosting glute and quad strength, but it's not as effective as a sumo squat for targeting the adductor, or inner thigh, muscles.

How to do it: Start in a traditional squat stance with your feet about shoulder-width apart and toes pointed forward. Take a step to the side with your right foot until your stance is about 1 metre wide, or wider than hip width.

Angle your toes out and away around 45 degrees laterally, rotating at the hip.

Move your hips back slightly and bend your knees as you lower your body into a squat position. Keep your core engaged, and eyes forward, throughout the movement. Lower until your thighs are parallel to the floor. You can go lower or shorten the squat if parallel is too low or if you can't maintain your leg alignment.

Pause in the squat position for a few seconds. Then, engaging your glutes, press up to standing, driving up through your heels.

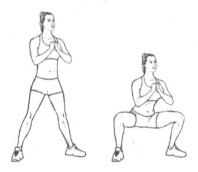

What are we working? Quadriceps, Gluteal muscles, Hips, Hamstrings, Calves, Inner thighs

Plank Rotations

The plank rotation activates the deep abdominal muscles and helps to tighten and stabilise your core. This exercise can help you improve balance, boost your endurance and increase core strength.

How to do it: Place yourself in a plank position with a straight body from head to toes. Tighten your abs and glutes to hold up your body. Lift one arm up towards the ceiling, slowing rotating your body in the same direction as you do so. Hold for 1–3 seconds, return slowly, and repeat on the other side to count one repetition. If you want to challenge yourself, you can do this exercise with weights.

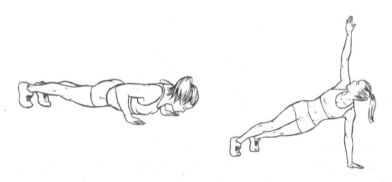

Dumbbell RDLs (Romanian Deadlifts)

Incorporating dumbbell RDLs into your workout routine can be really beneficial as these exercises are great for improving hip extension strength and building up muscle mass in your glutes and hamstrings. They can also help to enhance overall hip mobility, which is helpful as we go through menopause and midlife when we are potentially more prone to falls and hip fractures.

How to do it: Stand with your feet hip-width apart and slightly bend your knees. Take dumbbells in each hand and place them in front of your hips with your palms facing your thighs. As you send your hips back, keep your spine in a neutral position and squeeze your shoulder blades together.

Keep sending your hips back and push your bum back as if you were shutting a cupboard with your glutes. With your chin tucked and shoulders squeezed, take the dumbbells following the line of your leg to halfway down on your shin. Drive up through the glutes as you come back up to standing still, following the line of your legs.

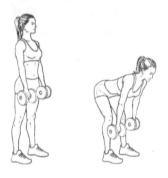

What are we working? Glutes, Lower back, Hamstrings

Good Mornings
Same technique as above but with no weights. Place your hands lightly behind your head with elbows facing out.

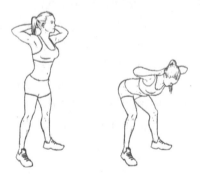

Press Ups
Press ups are an excellent way to strengthen the upper body, engaging the triceps, pectoral muscles and shoulders, as well as improving the lower back and core by engaging the abs. They are

a convenient and easy exercise that can be done anywhere without the need for any equipment, and you can begin at any level and progress as you build strength.

Release Press Ups

This is where you release at the bottom of the press up before going back up. These are the best press ups to begin with as you release the load of your bodyweight, which in turn can make it easier to power yourself back up and gradually build chest muscles. You will then progress to kneeling press ups when you feel more confident.

Knee Press Ups

These are press ups that you execute in a half position with your knees resting on the ground, rather than you whole body being used.

How to do it: Assume an all-fours position, then engage your core by contracting your abs and pulling your belly button towards the spine. Breathe in as you gradually lower yourself to the floor by bending your elbows until they form a 90-degree angle. Keep your forehead up and ensure that your chest area is positioned between your hands. As you exhale, contract your chest muscles and push yourself back up through your hands.

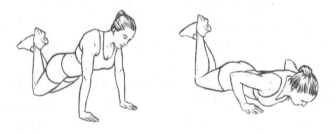

What are we working? Triceps, Pectorals, Shoulders

Full Press Ups

Once you have built up strength in your upper body you can progress to full press ups.

How to do it: Assume a plank position. Engage your core by contracting your abs and pulling your belly button towards the spine. Breathe in as you gradually lower yourself to the floor by bending your elbows until they form a 90-degree angle. Keep your forehead up and ensure that your chest area is positioned between your hands. As you exhale, contract your chest muscles and push yourself back up through your hands.

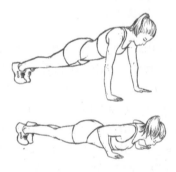

Bent Over Rows

One of the best back exercises to help build more muscle and strength is the bent over row. This exercise will promote better back posture, balance, core stability and strength. You'll need to engage your core throughout the entire movement, which can improve your strength and enhance your posture and balance. It benefits your core strength because your core is braced through-out the movement to stabilise your upper and lower back.

How to do it: Holding a dumbbell in each hand, bend your knees slightly and hinge at the hip so your upper body is almost parallel to the floor. Keep your core tight and your back straight as you row the weights up to your chest, almost as if you are putting them into your back pocket.

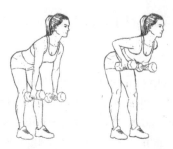

What are we working? Arms, Upper and Lower back, Shoulders, Core

Upright Rows

An upright row is an effective exercise to build strength in the shoulders and upper back. Strengthening your posterior chain is hugely beneficial for functional everyday life.

The exercise does have a reputation for causing injury, so a correct form is crucial.

How to do it: Stand with your feet shoulder-width apart, holding the dumbbells with an overhand grip down in front of you with your arms extended.

Begin to lift the dumbbells up, pulling through your elbows and keeping the weight close to your body as you go. Stop when your elbows are level with your shoulders and the dumbbell is at chest level. Keep your torso upright throughout the movement. Pause at the top, then return to the starting position.

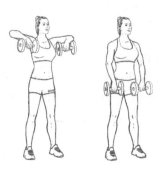

What are we working? Triceps, Pectorals, Shoulders

Bicep Curls

Bicep curls will help you build strength in the upper arm. Curls work the bicep muscles at the front of the upper arm and the muscles of the lower arm. We use these muscles whenever we pick something up, which is common throughout daily life, so it's important to train them.

How to do it: Begin by standing tall with your feet about hip-width apart. Keep your abdominal muscles engaged. Hold one dumbbell in each hand. Let your arms relax down at the sides of your body with palms facing inwards. Keeping your upper arms stable and shoulders relaxed, bend at the elbow and lift the weights so that the dumbbells approach your shoulders. Your elbows should stay tucked in close to your body. Exhale while lifting. Lower the weights to the starting position.

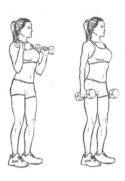

Bent Arm Lateral Raises

The bent arm lateral raise is an effective shoulder-strengthening movement. Performed regularly, this can help you develop stronger shoulders.

How to do it: Stand tall, a dumbbell in each hand. Arms are at your sides, palms facing in, elbows bent at a 90-degree angle. Position your feet roughly hip-distance apart. Check your posture – roll your shoulders back, engage your core and look straight ahead. Raise your arms to 90 degrees out to each side and pause. Breathe in as you lift. Pause and hold for a second at the top of the movement. Lower the weights, bringing your arms back to your sides. Breathe out as you lower the dumbbells.

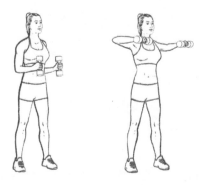

What are we working? Arms, Upper and Lower back, Shoulders, Core

Mountain Climbers

Mountain climbers are an effective bodyweight exercise that works many muscles. Your shoulder muscles, triceps, chest muscles, serratus anterior and abdominal muscles work mainly to support your body against gravity while holding a plank position. Your glutes, quads, hip flexors, hamstrings and calves are also recruited to move your legs during the exercise.

How to do it: Start on the floor on your hands and knees. Place your hands shoulder-distance apart and align your shoulders directly over your wrists. Step your right leg back into a high plank position, aiming to keep your body in a straight line from heel to head. Step your left leg back to meet your right leg in plank position. Keeping your neck in line with your spine, focus your gaze on a spot on the floor just in front of your hands. Using your abdominals, bend your right knee in towards your chest, then step it back into the plank position. Repeat with your left leg, bringing it towards your chest and then stepping it back.

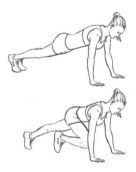

Tricep Extensions

The triceps extend, or straighten the elbow, and help the shoulder muscles to extend the arm. The overhead tricep extension is an excellent exercise to work this muscle. If the tricep extension is too hard, try the tricep kickbacks.

How to do it: Hold the dumbbell overhead by grasping the inside dumbbell plate surface with both hands. Slowly bend your elbows and lower the weight behind your head as far as you can. Ensure that your elbows are close to your ears, almost as if you are crushing your skull. Remember to keep your core engaged. The weight should follow the path of your spine. Then, at the lowest point, straighten your elbows and extend the weight back overhead. Hold the fully extended position for a moment, then repeat. Keep the movement slow and controlled.

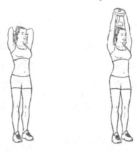

What are we working? Triceps, Shoulders, Core

Tricep Kickbacks

The tricep kickback is an excellent exercise to work the tricep and offers a variation to the tricep overhead. It can help work each tricep individually or unilaterally, creating more balance as the extension may see your stronger arm overcompensating for your weaker arm.

How to do it: Hold a dumbbell in each hand with your palms facing in towards each other, keeping your knees bent slightly. Engage your core and maintain a straight spine as you hinge forward at the waist, bringing your torso almost parallel to the floor. Keep your upper arms close to your body and your head in line with your spine, tucking your chin in slightly. On an exhale, engage your triceps by straightening your elbows. Hold your upper arms still, only moving your forearms during this movement. Pause here, then inhale to return the weights to the starting position.

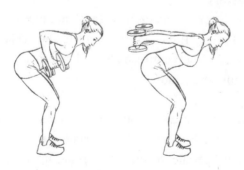

Overhead Presses

It's important to keep the muscles in your upper body conditioned and mobile. These muscles help you do everyday tasks, such as putting dishes up high or placing items overhead on a shelf. Keep your upper body in shape by including the overhead press, sometimes called the shoulder press, in your programme.

How to do it: Stand with your feet shoulder-width apart. Grab a pair of dumbbells and hold them at shoulder height. Make sure your spine is in a neutral position and you have a little bend in the knee. With palms facing inwards, drive the dumbbells overhead, then lower them slowly. Repeat this movement for your desired number of repetitions.

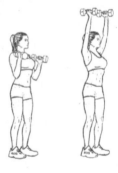

What are we working? Triceps, Shoulders, Lower back, Core

Squat Thrusters

Thrusters are a compound exercise that combines the squat with the overhead press. This is a very complete and versatile exercise that strengthens your entire body and improves your aerobic fitness, stamina and endurance.

How to do it: Stand with your feet shoulder-width apart and hold your dumbbells in front of your shoulders. Squat down until your thighs are parallel to the floor. Stand up and extend your arms over your head. Bend your arms, return to the starting position, and repeat the exercise.

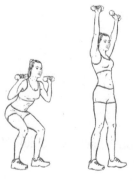

What are we working? Quads, Hamstrings, Glutes, Shoulders

Renegade Rows

The renegade row exercise focuses explicitly on the upper back muscles and the core. This is particularly beneficial for improving balance and coordination.

How to do it: Place the dumbbells on the floor with the handles parallel to each other and spaced about shoulder-width apart. Begin in a tabletop position with your hands under your shoulders and your knees under your hips, gripping a dumbbell in each hand. From here, step your feet back to enter a full plank position with your body straight from heels to head and your feet hip-width apart for stability. Inhale and shift your weight to one side, lifting the dumbbell in that hand towards your chest while keeping your hips and shoulders square to the floor. Exhale as you lift the weight and squeeze your shoulder blade towards your spine. Lower the weight back to the floor and repeat on the opposite side for one full repetition.

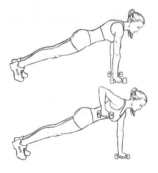

What are we working? Back, Shoulders, Biceps, Core

Dead Bugs
The dead bug exercise effectively strengthens and stabilises your core, spine and back muscles. This improves your posture and helps relieve and prevent lower back pain. You'll also improve balance and coordination.

How to do it: Lie on the mat with your arms extended straight over your chest so they form a perpendicular angle with your torso. Bend your hips and knees 90 degrees, lifting your feet from the ground. Your torso and thighs should form a right angle, as should your thighs and shins. This is the starting position. Engage your core, maintaining contact between your lower back and the mat. You want to ensure your spine maintains this steady and neutral position throughout the exercise. Keep your left arm and right leg exactly where they are, then slowly reach your right arm backwards, over your head and towards the floor, as you simultaneously extend your left knee and hip, reaching your left heel towards the floor. Move slowly and steadily as you swap sides, breathing in as you perform the extensions, avoiding any twisting or movement of your hips and abs. Stop the movement just before your arm and leg touch the ground.

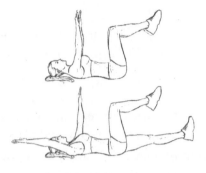

What are we working? Core, Deep abdominal muscles, Back, Spine

Plank Taps
Plank taps strengthen your core, glutes, arms, wrists and shoulders. This exercise helps to reduce lower back pain and improves your posture and flexibility. If the plank taps are too hard, try the renegade rows.

How to do it: Start in a plank position, with your wrists under your shoulders and your feet together. Engage your core and touch your left shoulder with your right hand. Return to plank and touch your right shoulder with your left hand and continue alternating sides until the set is complete. If full plank taps are too hard, you can drop to your knees and work from there.

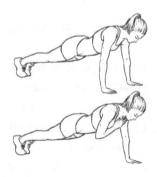

What are we working: Core, Arms

Walkouts

A walkout is a plank variation that works the core and shoulders and is often used as a good warm-up move as it gets the whole body moving.

How to do it: Start with your feet hip-width apart. Bending from your hips, reach for the ground and place your palms on the floor in front of your feet. Slowly shift your weight onto your hands and begin walking them forward until your body is in a straight line from your head to your heels, bracing your core and making sure your hands are directly under your shoulders in a shoulder, elbow, wrist line.

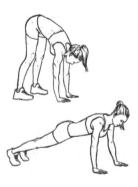

What are we working? Back, Shoulders, Core

Burpees

A good all-over cardio move to challenge the whole body.

How to do it: Start in a squat position with your knees bent, back straight and your feet together but not quite touching. Lower your hands to the floor in front of you. With your weight on your hands, kick your feet back so you're on your hands and toes and in a push-up position. Keeping your body straight from head to heels, do one press up. Remember not to let your back sag or to stick your butt in the air. Do a frog kick by jumping your feet back to their starting position. Stand and reach your arms over your head. Jump quickly into the air so you land back where you started. As soon as you land with knees bent, get into a squat position and do another repetition.

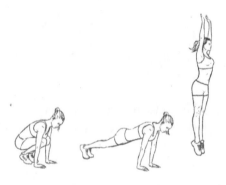

What are we working? Back, Shoulders, Core

Bikes

Bicycle crunches work your lower, middle and upper abs while strengthening your quads and hamstrings.

How to do it: Start by lying on the ground, with your lower back pressed flat into the floor. Place your hands lightly on the sides of your head; don't knit your fingers behind. Lift one leg just off the ground and extend it out. Lift the other leg and bend your knee towards your chest. As you do so, twist through your core, so the opposite arm comes towards the raised knee. You don't need to touch elbow to knee, instead focus on moving through your core as you turn your torso. Your elbow should stay in the same position relative to your head throughout – the turn that brings it closer to the knee comes from your core.

Lower your leg and arm at the same time, while bringing up the opposite two limbs to mirror the movement. Keep on alternating.

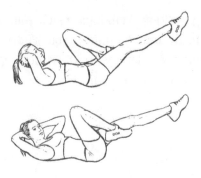

Twists

The twist is a great exercise to strengthen your core and shoulder strength. Although it looks easy, it takes a lot of effort and stability.

How to do it: In a sitting position, sit deep into the bones as you lift your feet from the floor, keeping your knees bent. Lift your chest up to the sky and straighten your spine at a 45-degree angle from the floor, creating a V-shape with your torso and thighs. Reach your arms straight out in front, interlacing your fingers or clasping your hands around the weight, if using. Use your abdominals to twist to the right, then back to centre, and then to the left.

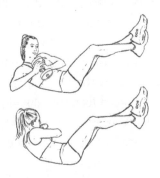

What are we working? Core, Shoulders, Obliques

Jackknives

A great exercise to work and challenge the obliques and deeper abdominal muscles.

How to do it: Lengthen your body on your mat and lie flat, neutralising your lower back by drawing your belly button into your spine and tilting your pelvis to the ceiling. For alternating jackknives stretch your legs out long and reach your arms above your head. Hover your arms and legs a few inches off the mat. Take a deep breath and on your exhale, lift your head and pull the opposite arm and leg up into a V-shape (lift roughly 30–45 degrees away from the mat). On the next rep, reach for the opposite leg to the arm you have raised. On your lift, keep your legs straight and your arms parallel to your thighs. Lower back down to your starting position. For full jackknives, take a deep breath and on the exhale lift your head and both arms into a V-shape to meet the shins (as pictured).

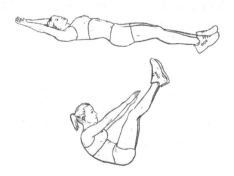

What are we working? Upper and Lower abdominals, Obliques

Chest Presses

This is one of the best chest exercises for building upper body strength and can help with daily activities, such as carrying shopping, reaching for objects and pushing heavy doors.

How to do it: Lie on your back holding two dumbbells at chest height. Press up until your arms are fully extended. Slowly lower back to the starting position, imagining you have a sheet of glass under you as you lower your elbows towards the floor steadily and controlled before powering the dumbbells back up to full extension.

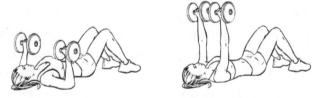

What are we working? Arms, Chest, Shoulders

Push Presses
This is a great exercise that increases upper and lower body strength and power. By using this movement with the explosive push needed, you can help build stability and balance. It will also help build strength in your shoulders and enable you to feel more confident in lifting heavy objects overhead or having to retrieve objects from cupboards up high.

How to do it: Standing with your feet at hip width and holding dumbbells up in front of your shoulders, bend your knees slightly and lower down just a bit. Then, quickly stand up and simultaneously press the dumbbells up overhead. Keeping your glutes and core engaged will stabilise your spine.

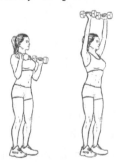

What are we working? Lower and Upper body, Glutes, Pecs, Triceps, Deltoids, Quadriceps, Lower back muscles

Dumbbell Swings

Dumbbell swings may not be one of the most common exercises, but they can be highly effective and a great way to improve the strength and stability of your core. Keep making sure your spine is in a neutral position as this will help if you have experienced back pain in the past and will prevent any reoccurance.

How to do it: Place your feet a little wider than shoulder-width apart. Hold the dumbbell with both hands and do a squat so that you can bring the weight between your legs while keeping your arms fully extended. Swing the weight between your legs. After the weight reaches behind you, thrust your hips forward and drive the weight upward towards your chest. Arc the weight back down to the starting position and repeat.

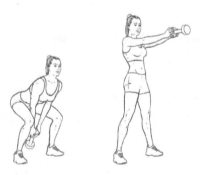

What are we working? Glutes, Thighs, Core muscles

Reverse Flys

A great but challenging exercise to help you build strength in your upper back, shoulders and core.

How to do it: Stand with feet shoulder-width apart, holding dumbbells at your sides. Press the hips back in a hinge motion, bringing your chest forward and almost parallel to the floor. Let the weights hang straight down (palms facing each other) while maintaining a tight core, straight back and slight knee bend. Raise both arms out to your side on an exhale. Keep a soft bend in your elbows. Squeeze the shoulder blades together as you pull them towards the spine. Lower the weight back to the start position as you inhale. Avoid hunching your shoulders, and keep your chin tucked to maintain a neutral spine during the exercise.

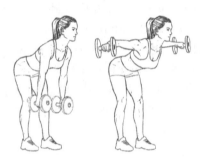

What are we working? Back, Shoulders

Dumbbell Snatches

The dumbbell snatch is a great all-over body move to help you target multiple muscle groups and build strength and power.

How to do it: Stand shoulder-width apart with a dumbbell on the floor between your feet. Keep your shoulders back, chest out and eyes facing straight ahead. Ensure your back is straight. Push your hips back (hinge your hips) and bend your knees into a squat position. Be mindful you aren't just bending over, so you are protecting your lower back. With a straight left arm, grab the dumbbell with an overhand grip. You should not have to reach far ahead or behind to grab the dumbbell. Drive down into your heels and stand up quickly (explosively) using your legs and glutes – your feet may leave the ground. Using the momentum of your lower body, begin to raise the dumbbell vertically in a straight line. It should be kept close to your body. As the dumbbell comes up to your shoulder height, begin to pull the dumbbell backward towards your chest and flip your elbow so it's now below the dumbbell. Press upward with the dumbbell – similar to an upward punching motion – so that it's above your head with a straight arm. To lower the weight, bend your elbow outward and down (parallel to your shoulder) and slowly lower the weight back down to your side. Then bend your knees and hinge your hips to lower the weight back to the ground.

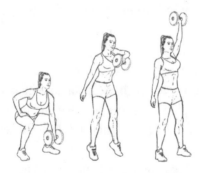

What are we working? Glutes, Hamstrings, Quads, Shoulders, Core

Hip Thrusts

This is a great exercise to help you build strength and stability by focusing on getting you to engage muscles in the hip, buttocks and quadriceps. If you have had a diagnosis of osteopenia or osteoporosis, this will help you target low bone density in the hips and femur bones, align your knee joints and promote better balance.

How to do it: Lie on your back with knees bent, feet planted firmly on the floor. Engage and brace the core and press your heels into the floor, driving your hips upwards and towards your head. Pause at the top, squeezing the glutes and lowering down, ensuring your core is engaged.

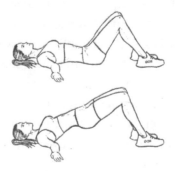

What are we working? Glutes, Hamstrings, Quads

Bear Taps
Plank variations are great when it comes to keeping your core strong, minimising lower back pain and maximising performance. The bear plank is a core bodyweight exercise that focuses on strengthening the muscles that stabilise your spine.

How to do it: Begin on your hands and knees with your feet flexed and toes on the floor. Your weight should be evenly distributed across your fingers, palms and the heels of your hand. Engage your glutes to slightly tuck in your tailbone. Contract your abdominals by taking a full breath and drawing them in as if you're bracing for a punch. The bottom of your ribs should move slightly towards your pelvis. Lift your knees about 2–3cm so that they're floating just above the ground. Keep your chin and head in a neutral position, with your gaze fixed on the floor directly beneath your head. Breathe in and out in a controlled manner while maintaining your brace. As you exhale, lift your right hand to tap your left shoulder. Ensure that your core is strong and you avoid arching the spine or dropping your stomach. On the next breath, place your right hand to the floor and lift your left hand to tap your right shoulder. Continue for the desired amount of reps.

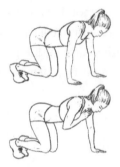

What are we working? Core, Shoulders

Side Shuffles
This exercise is a great way to strengthen your lower body, plus it adds a little cardio into your existing workout programme. It is also great for balance and agility as you are moving laterally.

How to do it: Make sure you have space on either side of you. Facing forwards, take tiny sprint steps from side to side. Try not to bend through the back so you don't strain.

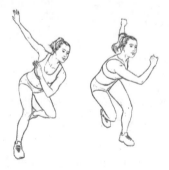

Star Steps/Jumps
This exercise can challenge your glutes, quads and hip flexors. It

is a compound movement, so it pretty much works every muscle in your body.

How to do it: Make sure you have space on either side. Facing forwards, take tiny steps with one leg out to the side and lift both arms. Repeat on the other side. If doing jumps – jump out both legs at the same time and lift your arms overhead.

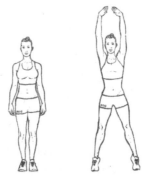

Isolation Movements

Isolation exercises tackle one specific muscle group or joint. Although simple, they are best used once you have built good overall strength. An example of an isolation exercise is the bicep curl, as you are only challenging the biceps on their own.

Kneel Ups

Kneel to standing is an exercise that will help target the glutes and build stability, balance and mobility.

How to do it: Get into the kneeling position. For the bodyweight version, place your hands behind your head in a prisoner hold (this will make it harder). Step up with your left leg while keeping weight on your right knee. Get up into the standing position, driving through your left heel. Bring your right foot forward and stand up nice and tall. Repeat on the other side. For the weighted version you can have a dumbbell in each hand or hold one dumb-bell in front of you. This will add resistance and weight to the move, again making it harder to execute.

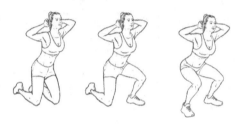

Arm Circles

This exercise will encourage you to not only use your arms but also your core.

It can really work on shaping the muscles in your shoulders and arms and can be a lovely way to get moving without too much pressure or stress on the body.

How to do it: Place your feet firmly on the ground and engage your core. Take your arms out to the side and extend away from the body. Standing tall, make little circles forwards and backwards.

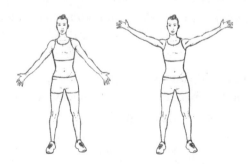

Punches

A great little heart rate raiser and core strengthener.

How to do it: Place your feet firmly on the ground and engage your core. Propel your hands forwards with clenched fists and punch out ahead.

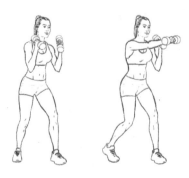

Front Raises

Great for building shoulder strength.

How to do it: Stand with your feet about shoulder-width apart. Let your arms hang in front of you with the dumbbells in front of the thighs (palms facing the thighs). Your back is straight, your feet are planted flat on the floor, and your core is engaged. Lift the weights upward while inhaling. Your arms are extended, palms facing down, with a slight bend in the elbows to reduce the stress on the joints. Pause briefly when your arms are horizontal to the floor. Lower the dumbbells to the starting position (at the thighs) with a slow and controlled motion while exhaling.

Alternating Front Raises

Raise each arm separately and individually. Once one arm is down, raise the other. This is one rep.

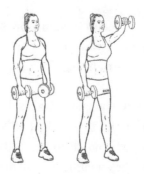

Stretches

Cat Cows
How to do it: Start on your hands and knees, making sure your wrists, elbows and shoulders are aligned. Tilt your pelvis back so that your tailbone sticks up. Your belly will drop down, but draw your belly button into your spine. Take your gaze gently up towards the ceiling without cranking your neck. Release the tops of your feet to the floor. Tip your pelvis forward, tucking your tailbone under. Draw your belly button towards your spine. Drop your head. Take your gaze to your belly button.

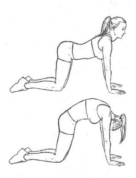

Bird Dogs
How to do it: Begin on all fours in the tabletop position. Place your knees under your hips and your hands under your

shoulders. Maintain a neutral spine by drawing your belly button into your spine. Draw your shoulder blades together. Raise your left arm and right leg, keeping your shoulders and hips parallel to the floor.

Lengthen the back of your neck and tuck your chin into your chest to gaze down at the floor. Hold this position for a few seconds, then lower back down to the starting position. Raise your right arm and left leg, holding this position for a few seconds. Return to the starting position.

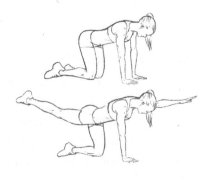

Thread the Needles

How to do it: Start on your hands and knees, walk your right hand forward and slide the left hand between the right knee and the right hand. Twist your torso to the right and rest your head on the mat. Stay in the pose for 30 seconds, return to neutral position, reverse hands, and repeat.

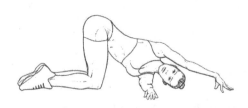

Hip Flexors
How to do it: Standing up tall, take a big step forward with your left foot and go into a lunge position, pointing your back foot so that your sole is facing up. Place your hands on your hips or on your forward knee. Tip your hips back so you can feel the stretch and hold for 20-30 seconds.

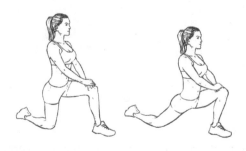

Piriformis Stretches
How to do it: Lie on your back with both knees bent and your feet flat on the floor. Put the ankle of the leg you intend to stretch on your opposite thigh near your knee. Use your hand to gently pull your thigh towards your body until you feel a gentle stretch around your hip. Hold for the desired time and repeat on the opposite leg.

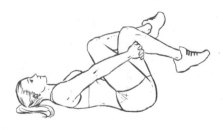

Chest and Bicep Stretches

How to do it: Interlace your fingers behind your back. Keep your hands at the base of your spine. Straighten your arms. Lift your arms as high as you can, letting your body bend forward.

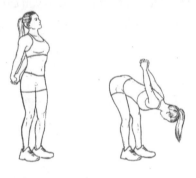

Tricep Stretches

How to do it: Stand straight with your feet hip-width apart. Lift and bend one arm until your hand is in the middle of the upper back. Grasp the elbow with the other hand and gently pull.

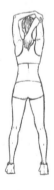

The Baby

How to do it: Lie on your back and hug your knees to your chest, or hold your feet and rock from side to side. This is great for the back to release and also helps with mobility in the hips. This move is often used in yoga or at the end of sessions to promote calm and relaxation.

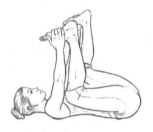

PART 4
Owning Your Recovery

Many women need help unravelling the myth and the fear that has become ingrained in them that a rest day or days off may hinder their progress. This couldn't be further from the truth. In fact, allowing yourself time to rest is a complete game changer in making a sustainable change to a fitter, calmer and stronger future, in particular for those struggling with joint aches and pains and motivation.

There are a number of ways in which we can help the body to recover and repair. Some, like stretching, are more obvious than others as we have been made aware of them. Allowing the body time to cool down after a workout can also be beneficial, but there are some less obvious recovery strategies that I am also keen to highlight.

Sleep is one of the most important elements in recovery, but sleep deprivation is one of the symptoms that I hear women are most affected by as they journey through and beyond menopause. This can be due to the night sweats you can experience or you may simply find yourself unsettled and restless for large periods in the night.

I have added a section on this with help from sleep expert Kathryn Pinkham as managing disrupted sleep is one of the things I would love you to take away with you after reading this book. It will really help you make fitness progress and strength gains.

We will also look at the importance of breathing correctly. This involuntary bodily function that most of us take for granted has many benefits and if we can unlock these it can be very powerful. It is an incredible free and useful tool for your recovery and this, alongside cold-water immersion, can also help manage any anxiety you may be experiencing, which in turn can disrupt sleep.

CHAPTER 13

How to Recover
After Your Workout

There are two types of recovery: active and passive. Both are equally important, and you can use one or the other at different times.

Active recovery
In its simplest form, this means working your muscle groups after exercise. This could be done on the same day or as your actual progress day. Active recovery would be achieved by going for a walk, doing some yoga, Pilates or swimming. If movement is important for you daily because it helps you mentally, then this style of recovery is more for you.

Passive recovery
This entails stillness or inactivity – you simply let your body rest while sitting or lying. Other forms of passive recovery are meditation, mindfulness and cold-water therapy.

You will enhance your well-being and find that your routine becomes more sustainable and achievable if you allow time for your mind and body to recover.

One of my favourite things to share is the power of reframing situations and thoughts. What if you were to consider renaming your rest days and started calling them progress days, would you make them a priority?

We want to avoid exercise-induced fatigue. If we keep putting our bodies under stress-induced exercise, this will lead to muscle fatigue and soreness. If you don't rest, you're likely to put yourself at an increased risk of injury, which is only going to see you having to take more rest days and time out.

The other benefit of resting is that it gives your body time to replenish much-needed energy stores. When we exercise, the body breaks down glycogen or energy to fuel our workouts. If you rest and recover you will come back fitter, calmer and stronger.

Progress days are therefore an important part of your toolkit. They help manage many of your symptoms of menopause and play a large role in ensuring your cortisol levels don't get too high.

Having discussed the long-term benefits of rest and recovery, let's focus on what to do immediately after a workout because there are a few steps you can take within the first couple of hours of finishing your session to help start the recovery process.

- **Stay hydrated**
  This may seem obvious, but it's often forgotten due to our busy lifestyles. Rehydration is important, especially after an intense and sweaty session. You should replace your fluid levels to improve your muscle flexibility, build strength and prevent muscle soreness.
- **Stretch**
  Make sure to always finish your workout with a stretch. This will help your heart rate gradually return to its normal resting state and relieve any stress in your muscles, preventing soreness and injury. Remember, your cool-down only needs to be 5 minutes long, but it can make a significant difference in how you feel the next day.

- **Protein-rich food**

  Aim to have a protein-rich meal within 1–2 hours of your workout or immediately after if you need it. This will help refuel and aid muscle recovery. It is really important to eat something sensible and avoid sugary snacks because these will not optimise recovery and will leave you feeling hungrier sooner as you dip after the initial rush.

- **Shower**

  It's important to remember to shower after a workout! If you're thinking of staying in your workout clothes for a bit, taking the time to rinse off will help prevent bacteria and yeast from building up on your skin. Many women experience irritated skin as they go through menopause or an increase in body odour. If you make time for a quick shower, it will decrease your risk of irritation and infection.[31]

It's important to stick to your post-fitness routine as much as possible, but if you're ever short on time or have other commitments, it's OK to deviate occasionally. Keep in mind that your body needs rest and recovery, so if you ever feel tired, ill or in pain after exercising, it's important to take a break. By allowing your body to fully recuperate, you'll be better prepared to perform at your best during your next workout.

What is DOMS?

Sore muscles after physical activity, known as delayed onset muscle soreness (DOMS), can occur when you start a new exercise programme, change your exercise routine or increase the duration or intensity of your regular workouts. When muscles are required to work harder than they are used to or in a different way, we cause microscopic damage to the muscle fibres, resulting in muscle soreness or stiffness. It is very common but as your muscles begin to build and change, you are likely to experience fewer DOMS occurrences.

If you don't rest and allow recovery time, you may notice some of the following signs, which would indicate that it might be time to take a longer rest between workouts.[32]

- **Sore muscles**
  While it's normal to feel sore after exercise, persistent soreness is a red flag. It means your muscles haven't recovered from past workouts.
- **Fatigue**
  Pay attention to extreme exhaustion. If you feel spent, let your body rest.
- **Pain**
  Muscle or joint pain that doesn't go away might be a sign of an overuse injury.
- **Emotional changes**
  When you're physically burnt out, hormones like serotonin and cortisol become imbalanced. This can cause changes like irritability, crankiness and mood swings.
- **Sleeping issues**
  High levels of cortisol and adrenalin can make it hard to get quality sleep.
- **Reduced performance**
  If your normal routine feels difficult, or if you stop seeing progress, take a progress day.

This kind of muscle pain should not be confused with any other kind of pain that you might experience during exercise, such as the acute, sudden or sharp pain of an injury, like a muscle strain or sprain.

CHAPTER 14

Sleep

Sleep, or lack of it, is something that women going through menopause can relate to, and sleep deprivation is remarkably unforgiving.

Sleep is part of our recovery, and lack of sleep can contribute to poor health. It can also have a significant impact on our mental health, which may already be at risk as we transition through menopause. Sleep quality before and after exercise is important. Researchers suspect that it is the deep sleep that helps improve athletic performance because this is the time when growth hormone is released. Growth hormone is a small protein that is made by the pituitary gland and more is produced at night. It stimulates the growth of bone and cartilage, muscle growth and repair, and fat burning.[33]

Disruptions to your sleep pattern – whether chronic or acute – can promote an unhealthy increase in our cortisol, or stress, levels and impact our hunger hormones, which can also contribute to overeating.

The National Sleep Foundation recommends that adults get between 7 and 9 hours of sleep per night. Increasing sleep time by 1 hour per night is like getting an entire extra night's worth of sleep over the course of a week.[34]

How can we improve our chances of a good night's sleep?

It's important to calm the mind before bed, so consider switching off your mobile phone an hour before bedtime and practising relaxation techniques.

Making sure you eat well throughout the day, including plenty of protein in your diet. Additionally, taking magnesium glycinate as a supplement can improve sleep quality, reduce restless legs syndrome symptoms and make it easier to fall asleep. We'll dive more into supplements later in the book (see Chapter 18).

Remember not to worry about sleep, as worrying only makes things worse. If you find yourself feeling stressed and awake in bed, try leaving the bedroom and doing something relaxing, like reading a book downstairs.

When you feel tired, return to bed and give yourself a chance to rest.

Kathryn Pinkham of The Insomnia Clinic offers these top tips to improve sleep in menopause: [35]

• **CBT**

CBT-I is recommended by the NHS as it has repeatedly been shown to help menopausal women improve their sleep, using techniques that will increase their body's natural drive to sleep better and also reduce the worry and anxiety attached to poor sleep. I focus on exploring the connection between the way we think, the things we do and how we sleep. A trained CBT-I provider helps to identify thoughts, feelings and behaviours that are contributing to the symptoms of insomnia. You can refer yourself directly to an NHS talking therapies service without a referral from a GP. Your GP can also refer you if you would prefer.

- **Don't spend too long in bed**

  The first thing we do when we can't sleep is to start going to bed earlier to try and increase our opportunities for sleeping. Reduce the amount of time you spend in bed, go to bed later, and get up earlier. This will encourage your body's natural sleep drive to kick in. By reducing the time you spend in bed, you will crave more sleep, fall asleep faster and find your quality of sleep will improve.

- **Set a wake time and stick to it, regardless of how badly you have slept**

  By getting up early you will train your body clock to associate mornings with being awake. Staying in bed, and dozing, often results in grogginess and low mood, so instead get up, have a cuppa, and get some fresh air and exercise rather than trying to catch up on lost sleep.

- **Stop clock watching**

  If you are waking from hot flushes, then it is very tempting to look at the clock with each wakening to monitor how little sleep you are getting. However, this increases the pressure to fall back to sleep and makes it less likely. Set your alarm for the morning then avoid looking at the time again.

- **Don't lie in bed awake**

  If you can't get to sleep after a hot flush or can't fall asleep, get out of bed. The longer we lie in bed trying to fall back to sleep, the more frustrated we get. This, in turn, means we begin to subconsciously relate bed to feeling stressed and being awake rather than asleep and it makes it more likely that this pattern will continue. Leave the bedroom and do something relaxing like reading a book downstairs, then when you are tired, go back to bed.

- **Don't worry about it**

  Identify that you might be worried, but understand that worry can trigger more adrenalin. Learn to notice the worries rather than engaging with them. Challenge them by raising your belief that you will cope even though it might be hard.

Follow the above tips to give yourself the best possible chance of sleeping well, but outside of that, accept that sleep is not the only thing you can do to feel better. Try to leave a bad night behind you and focus on the day ahead. Go for a walk, get some fresh air and eat healthily to improve energy levels, rather than just focusing on sleep.

CHAPTER 15

Alternative Recovery Methods

There are many ways in which you can optimise your rest, recovery and progress days. You may opt for the more traditional methods like yoga, walking or simple stretching, but many people are using alternatives, like cold-water swimming and breathwork.

However you choose to recover is of course up to you, but adding these other methods into your weekly practice can be hugely beneficial. They are also free and easy to use and once you get the hang of them, they can help across all areas of your well-being practice.

Cold water

Taking a post-workout plunge in an ice-water bath or standing in a cold shower seems to be more common these days. I have found cold water a complete game-changer in my own journey. Not only do I feel it has helped me recover quicker but it has helped manage my anxiety, which has been one of my most significant symptoms. Better known as cold-water immersion or cryother-apy, it is thought to enable faster recovery and reduce muscle pain and soreness after intense training sessions.[36] Cold water can be literally shocking, mentally and physically.

Not only does it benefit recovery from workouts, but cold-water exposure done safely can offer many other benefits, in particular for women going through menopause. There is still much research to be done, but there is overwhelming positive anecdotal evidence from many women suggesting it has helped them. Mostly noted is the reduction in stress and anxiety, boosting immunity, improving circulation and skin, and relieving joint aches and pains.

Anna Gough, an expert in the field of breathwork and cold-water therapy says:

> *Plunging into an ice bath or getting yourself wet and wild outside in the extreme temperatures of mid-winter is being seen as the latest 'fad', but let's not forget that this is how our ancestors would bathe. We're evolving, especially since Covid, and looking for more primal, natural ways of igniting our inner resilience and, in turn, boosting our physical and emotional health.*

> *Cold water can be a most effective tool in bringing some balance and calm within many people's systems – both mind and body. It can also reduce stress and anxiety due to the increase in feel-good hormones and neurotransmitters once you immerse yourself in the cold.*

The British Medical Journal has also published a study showing how cold-water therapy can reduce depression and how, if done regularly, it could potentially help people come off their antidepressant medication.[37]

Some of us can feel an overwhelming amount of aches and

pains due to a build-up of inflammation in the body as we go through menopause and while it may sound a little scary, the cold-shock factor throws us into a fight or flight response, releasing stress hormones including noradrenaline and endorphins, which have an analgesic effect, helping to ease those nagging pains.

Adding this to the mix with movement and exercise gives us a boost of dopamine, the body's feel-good chemical, and this coupled with the euphoria of being connected with the outdoors, if cold-water swimming, contributes and supports us greatly while bringing in a lasting sense of achievement and calm.

If you wanted to try this form of recovery or use it for all the other benefits it may offer, here's how you can do it at home:

Ice bath

You can use your bath at home to perform cold-water therapy. Some people like to add ice, but equally you could just use the cold water from your tap. If you do use ice, fill the bath, pour in the ice and let it sit for a few minutes.

Cold shower

Many women expose themselves to a few minutes in a cold shower, which is more accessible and controllable. I advise starting with warm water and slowly taking the temperature down. You can make it colder gradually over time.

Outdoor cold-water swim

Some people who have access to larger pools of water, such as outdoor pools or lakes, highlight the added benefits of cold-water immersion in natural surroundings. In fact, this is how I got into it and without doubt has an added healing effect.

Safety

Be mindful that exposure to cold temperatures may result in hypothermia. Always consult with a doctor before practising cold-water therapy and remove yourself from the cold water if you experience numbness, tingling, pain or discomfort.

Cold-water immersion can cause serious cardiac stress and has resulted in heart attacks and death. Exposure to cold water can also affect your blood pressure, circulation and heart rate.

Breathwork

Anna Gough also highlights the power of breathwork, which is an integral part of recovery. Breathing is an easy activity; you even do it unconsciously. Everyone breathes because humans need it to survive, but did you know that deep breathing is a great stress reliever that can benefit your recovery?

Deep breathing is a specialised form of breathing used to help individuals with anxiety and stress. It can help with sleep quality, building resilience and improving your overall state of health.

Deep breathing is also an effective way of easing the body out of exercise mode and aid recovery effectively after exercise. Breathing exercises help to relax you, and they also encourage muscle repair and recovery. In the practices shared in the 30-Day Plan, you will learn how to become calmer, more present and conscious of your body and become more aware of 'you' in the moment. This is the gift of breathwork and it's accessible 24/7.

Try if you can to make a commitment to just a few minutes each day to tune into your breathing, which is great for your well-being, especially during menopause.

Summary

- Rest is a key part of a sustainable fitness programme.

- Look at your rest days as progress days and make them non-negotiable.

- There are two types of recovery: active and passive. Both are equally important.

- DOMS (delayed onset muscle soreness) is common when you begin a new fitness routine or change your exercise. It should not be confused with an acute or sharp pain.

- If we don't rest and recover, we can leave ourselves at risk of raised cortisol levels, which can have a detrimental effect on our hormone health and lead to weight gain around the middle.

- Sleep can play a huge role in your recovery and it is really important to take time to look at how you can improve this in order to give yourself the best chance of progress in a fitness routine as you go through menopause.

PART 5

Owning Your Nutrition

You can't out train a bad diet.

I have made it my mission to educate myself about how and what it is we need to do to nourish ourselves at this time so that we can truly thrive.

Like with exercise, people have differing opinions on how to nourish their bodies and there is a lot of misinformation and so many different trends that it can be overwhelming, confusing and cause anxiety around food for many women in midlife. Exercise and ensuring you have a nourishing, wholesome diet go hand in hand, and we need to balance the two.

It may all seem complicated and impossible to know the best way, but if you implement a few key food principles, which we will look at in this section, then you can learn to work out what is best for you and keep it simple, while ensuring you nourish and fuel your body.

It is important to remember that we are all different and our journeys are unique. I am going to help you create your own individual toolbox based on your experiences and goals in order to help you find a sustainable, achievable and manageable way to move and nourish your body.

CHAPTER 16

Weight Loss

We are living in a society where we all want a quick fix. We want maximum gain with minimum effort. This is where the conversations around keto, low carb, low fat, juicing, intermittent fasting and every other crazy way we are told to nourish our bodies need to stop. These ways of eating may have worked for some women at some point in their lives, but they are not going to be a sustainable or suitable prescription for every woman, especially as she goes through menopause.

Some women need to lose weight because they have been told to by their GP or health-care provider. If we are at risk of Type 2 diabetes and heart disease, then this must be addressed with a sensible, supported approach, which we will do in the 30-Day Plan.

It is also okay to want to lose weight, but only if you need to. In Chapter 5, I talked about reframing your why and mindset because we often put unrealistic expectations on ourselves. Instead, we must start embracing our changing bodies as we go through this transition. It's no good chasing your 30-year-old self because you will put your body through unnecessary stress and make unsustainable choices.

HRT and weight

I have seen many women who have started HRT and wrongly assumed that this will prevent further weight gain. While this could make sense that now we are replacing the oestrogen, we have to remember that weight gain is influenced by a number of things. Taking HRT doesn't replace the need for exercise and the lifestyle changes you must consider making to lose or maintain weight.

As we transition through menopause and our hormones decline, our bodies decide to recognise these declining ovarian oestrogen levels and look elsewhere for the hormone in a weak form of oestrogen produced by fat cells. In response, the body tries to create a reserve of oestrogen in its fat cells, which tend to build up fat stores around the middle area.

Lower testosterone levels during perimenopause and menopause can also slow your metabolism, making it harder to shift fat. Genetic factors might also play a role in menopause weight gain. If your parents or other close relatives carry extra weight around the abdomen, you will likely do the same.

I am asked by women daily for help managing their diet to try and alleviate many of their symptoms, and I don't ever want to overcomplicate it.

Here are five questions to ask yourself:

1. Are you reducing or quitting drinking alcohol?
2. Are you reducing your intake of refined sugars and processed food?
3. Are you eating three balanced meals daily – not juicing, restricting, fasting, or the like?
4. Is your plate full of protein, carbohydrates and fats?
5. Have you cut back on snacking?

If you have answered YES to all these questions, you are moving sensibly, resting enough and you are still struggling, then it would be advisable to seek further advice from your GP or a dietician.

Cortisol and the role it plays in weight gain in menopause

Cortisol is a vital hormone that plays many roles in our body. It is released in response to stress, and over time elevated levels can contribute to weight gain, especially around your abdomen.

I see many women worrying about cortisol levels having a negative impact on their weight. It is important to know that we do need cortisol, so in order to ensure we can manage this correctly, we must think about adding movement and implementing a diet that can help our body manage any unnecessary stress.

This is why rest days and recovery days are an important part of the programme. If we don't get enough rest or allow ourselves and our body time to repair, we can risk raising our cortisol levels excessively. So, while exercise is non-negotiable at this time, we also have to remember that it shouldn't put stress on the body.

High levels of cortisol can also actually replicate many of the symptoms of menopause, such as fatigue, poor sleep, heart palpitations, anxiety, irritability, high blood pressure and weight gain, which could all be confused with menopause.

You can see from this how entwined our hormone health is with exercise and movement and how important it is to find the balance between exercise and rest in order to prevent any negative effects that will hinder progress.

HIGH CORTISOL SYMPTOMS

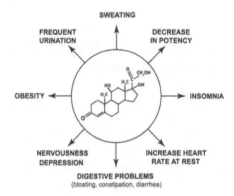

Weight and your metabolism

It's important to recognise that your metabolism is unique and so you need an individualised approach to your diet as you go through menopause. We will look at the factors that may be responsible for the changes happening to you in order to help you work out what your approach might be. It's not a one-size-fits-all approach.

- We know that eating a healthy and varied diet rich in fibre, complex carbohydrates, protein and healthy fat will lessen the impact of our symptoms as we go through menopause and fuel and nourish the exercise or movement we are doing.

- We know that improving our gut health to support our gut bacteria can have a significant impact at this time and foods high in fibre like vegetables, fruit, legumes and whole grains are great for your gut health.

- Some women have been misled into thinking that they are just eating more and exercising less, which is a little dismissive, generalised and unhelpful. I see many woman who are still active and eating healthily gain weight.

Sleep and how your weight may be affected

Lack of sleep can lead to increased appetite and this is something that affects a number of women. Midlife women transitioning through menopause and postmenopause are more likely to report sleep difficulties, with the rates of self-reported sleep difficulties ranging between 40 per cent and 56 per cent, compared to premenopausal women in the late-reproductive stage, who have rates of 31 per cent.[38]

Leptin and ghrelin are the hormones responsible for triggering this response.[39] Leptin is the appetite-regulating hormone released from fat cells. Ghrelin is the hormone that increases your appetite and plays a major role in body weight. When a person sleeps, leptin levels normally rise, subduing the need to eat by reassuring the brain that energy reserves are adequate for the time. However, sleep deprivation increases ghrelin levels, while at the same time lowering leptin levels in the blood.[40]

The lower levels of oestrogen in your body affect the amount of leptin your body produces, causing a decrease in leptin levels, while your ghrelin levels seem to rise, making it more difficult to keep the hunger hormones balanced.

The more body fat you have, the higher your leptin levels tend to be. Leptin is a hormone that decreases your appetite. Ghrelin is not affected by body fat and comes from your stomach. The hormone signals hunger and activates the brain's reward centre. This means that ghrelin is also responsible for the emotional hunger that causes us to eat those high-fat, high-carbohydrate foods.

These hormones do not work appropriately if you are overweight, binge eat or are in the dieting cycle. These two hormones become unbalanced because the brain becomes resistant to leptin (the appetite suppressant) due to restrictive eating. You must eat a balanced diet that includes high-quality foods to negate the imbalance.

Managing your blood sugar in menopause

It is crucial to understand the impact of menopause on blood sugar. Although this is not my area of expertise, I have made myself aware of the impact this can have on our overall health and well-being. Understanding this can help us comprehend the increased risk of Type 2 diabetes and midsection weight gain.

As someone with a sweet tooth, I had to work diligently to overcome my habit of indulging in sugary snacks. Moreover, I noticed an increase in snacking frequency entering this phase of life, likely due to changes in my blood sugar levels.

It is now clear to me how important it is to provide my body with proper nourishment and exercise throughout the day to prevent these dips and avoid making 'unhealthy' food choices that can lead to fatigue, exhaustion and weight gain.

Blood sugar, or the blood glucose level, is the amount of glucose found in the blood. Glucose is a simple carbohydrate found in bread, grains, fruit, dairy products and vegetables. Glucose is an important fuel for the body, but in high doses for any length of time, it can cause problems.

Insulin is a hormone produced in the pancreas that helps your body use glucose for energy; it then stores the remainder.[41] Oestrogen helps to optimise insulin but hormonal shifts play a major role in affecting blood sugar because oestrogen and progesterone, both of which are declining at this point, affect our insulin and how it works in the body.

Premenopausal women have increased insulin sensitivity (meaning their bodies use insulin effectively); however, after menopause and because of the reduction of oestrogen in the body, it appears that our body does not respond as well to insulin and, therefore, our blood sugar increases.

Relying on simple carbohydrates as our main calorie source can result in a rapid conversion into glucose that enters the bloodstream, causing a spike in blood sugar levels. To prevent this, the body produces excessive amounts of insulin, which can eventually lead to insulin resistance, where cells no longer respond to insulin. It is this insulin resistance that can lurk beneath two of the most common symptoms women experience during menopause: fatigue and weight gain.

If you are diagnosed with insulin resistance, the sooner you address it, the better, because you will be giving yourself a great opportunity to change your future with better nutrition.

CHAPTER 17

Why Gut Health Matters

Did you know that your gut is home to a vast network of bacteria, viruses and fungi called microbes and that these microbes play a significant role in our body's health, particularly as we enter menopause?

Katie Skrine, a qualified nutritionist, says the role of our digestive system (or gut as it is often referred to) isn't just to digest food and absorb nutrients from the food we eat. It is responsible for clearing out old hormones, making specific vitamins (K & B12), defending against pathogens (diseases) and influencing our mood, brain function and body weight.

We therefore need to do everything we can to ensure it is working at an optimal level. This means balancing the good bacteria, which can be out of balance from the foods we eat, the alcohol we drink and the antibiotics we overconsume – all of which can lead to hormonal disturbances, inflammation and poor well-being.

If we enhance our digestive health, then we have a better chance of metabolising and modulating our body's circulating oestrogen, which can help to avoid unwanted perimenopausal symptoms such as low mood, anxiety, poor sleep, brain fog, aching joints and so on.

Signs your gut could be imbalanced

- constipation
- diarrhoea
- gas
- bloating
- reflux (acid in the back of the throat)
- poor skin
- low mood
- extreme tiredness
- weight gain

If you have tried tweaking your diet but continue to experience many of these symptoms, please see your healthcare provider to rule out anything else.

There are many ways you can help support your gut microbiome. By making minor, sustainable tweaks, you can start to see an improvement in many of your symptoms.

Essential foods to boost your gut health

Add	What	Benefit
Fibre (soluble)	Oats, fruits (figs, kiwis, pears, apples), carrots and beans	Great for maintaining healthy cholesterol and feeding our gut bacteria.
Fibre (insoluble)	Whole grains, nuts, seeds, cauliflower and legumes	Helps bulk up stools and increases motility in the gut.
Prebiotics	Onions, leeks, garlic, asparagus, mushrooms, green beans, chicory, beetroot, green bananas, nuts and grains	Feeds the good bacteria.
Probiotics	Fermented foods, such as kefir, live yoghurt, miso, kimchi, sauerkraut and kombucha	Populates your gut with good bacteria.

| Plants | Aim for 30 different coloured plant foods per week – including all herbs, spices, nuts, seeds, beans, fruits and veggies | Plant-based foods contain lots of fibre as well as vitamins, minerals, antioxidants and phytonutrients, all of which we need in abundance as our bodies mature and hormones fluctuate. They will help protect against heart disease, obesity, high blood pressure, diabetes and some cancers. Your gut loves plant-based foods and they will support your hormone balance, immunity and mood. |

30 different plant foods a week

Katie Skrine goes on to highlight that it may sound daunting to consume 30 different plant foods in a week, so below is an idea of how you can achieve this.

Vegetables	1. asparagus
	2. beetroot
	3. butternut squash
	4. sweet potato
	5. courgettes
	6. carrots
	7. cabbage
	8. red pepper
	9. red onion
	10. broccoli
Legumes	11. chickpeas
	12. kidney beans
	13. adzuki beans
	14. butterbeans
	15. brown lentils
Whole grains	16. quinoa
	17. brown rice
	18. oats
	19. barley
	20. wheatberries

Nuts and seeds	21. sunflower seeds
	22. peanuts
	23. chia seeds
	24. pistachios
	25. cashews
Fruits	26. raspberries
	27. apples
	28. kiwis
	29. dates
	30. bananas

Implementing the above will have a significant impact on your symptoms. It would be worth noting any changes you experience so you can see how beneficial this way of eating is alongside your exercise plan.

Katie works with many women who have found that they are experiencing more constipation; this is a regular occurrence at this time due to the decline of oestrogen, which can slow the colon down. It can also be a result of not drinking enough water, which will affect the consistency of your stools.

Specific foods to relieve constipation and improve gut motility

- cooked beetroot
- kiwis
- strawberries and raspberries
- carrots (skin on)
- flaxseeds – use a combination of whole and ground
- chia seeds
- 1 apple a day
- drink 2 litres of water throughout the day (including herbal teas)

Ways to beat the bloat through perimenopause and menopause

Properly chewing your food and avoiding processed foods with inflammatory ingredients are key steps to improving digestion and avoiding the bloat that many of us can experience as our hormones fluctuate.

If you look to incorporate whole grains, plant-based foods and fibre into your diet, these will be instrumental in helping. It is worth noting a few things that can affect any bloating you may be experiencing:

- Be mindful of how much you drink during meals and steer clear of fizzy drinks.
- Try to drink your fluids around your meals rather than at the same time.
- Aim to be consistent with your meal times and try to have a 4–5 hour gap between meals in order to allow your gut to digest meals properly.
- If you are eating protein at every meal, you will not only avoid bloating, but you will be able to sustain that gap and potentially have less of the afternoon slump if this is something you experience.
- Try to avoid eating late at night. I will encourage you to have a period of 12 hours overnight where you don't eat to allow your gut time to rest.
- Chewing gum and artificial sweeteners can also contribute to bloating, so it's best to avoid them.

In Chapter 15 I talked about alternative recovery methods and breathwork. This, alongside rest and sufficient sleep each night, can further support your digestive system and potentially help with bloating.

If you are experiencing continual bloating or any of the red flags indicated below, please see your doctor to rule out anything more sinister.

- blood in your stools
- unexplained or prolonged bloating
- IBS symptoms that last longer than 3 weeks
- a change in bowel habits

CHAPTER 18

How to Fuel Your Body So It Can Thrive

Are you one of those people who have been cutting out important nutrients or restricting your diet to achieve a certain look or feel? How many different diets have you experimented with? How many times have you counted calories or restricted your intake just to feel better?

The truth is, many of us have forgotten the basics of healthy eating. I work with clients who under-eat and make poor choices when they do eat. Food is a positive and essential component of life that can help manage the symptoms of menopause.

I know that changing our beliefs about food can be a challenge, but let's focus on the key food groups we should be eating, how much we should be eating and how this might improve our relationship with food.

I started a new position as Headteacher at a special school. Although I've been at the school for a long time, it's been a huge step up to take overall responsibility. It seemed a bit crazy to start exercising and managing my diet choices at such a stressful time, but it has been the best thing I could have done. I feel so much healthier, I am sleeping better and don't have the sluggish feeling I had in the morning. I am going to stick with cutting out sugar, mindless snacking and minimise gluten. I'm adding one thing back at a time to see how I go. Thank you so much.

Jo

Macronutrients

Macronutrients are the key nutrients that provide your body with energy and the components it needs to maintain its structure and functions.

The three macronutrients are carbohydrates, protein and fat. They're needed in relatively larger amounts than other nutrients, hence the term 'macro'. Although there are recommended ranges for macronutrient intake, your needs vary based on your personal circumstances.

Protein

Protein is important for repairing and strengthening muscles and keeping your bones strong and healthy. A woman naturally begins to lose muscle mass and bone strength as she ages, mainly as a result of decreasing oestrogen levels during the menopause transition, so protein is essential.

Protein also influences the release of hormones that control appetite and food intake. It can help you feel fuller for longer, helping curb that temptation to snack.

If you already eat a diet that is rich in meat, fish, dairy and eggs you are doing a great job, but are you eating enough?

Perimenopausal women should be looking to eat around 1–1.2g of protein per kilogram of body weight per day (a little more if you're very active, work out a lot, have recently been ill or have a physically demanding job). So, a 70kg woman needs around 70–84g of protein a day, ideally split across meals as your body can't break down large amounts in one go.

Many midlife women are time-poor and the last thing they want is to be hung up on continually counting and weighing food. If you can make sure you have three protein-rich meals a day, you will likely be hitting your target. However, if you notice you are hungry soon after you have eaten or you have cravings within 3–4 hours of your last meal and an early evening dip, it may be an indication that you aren't getting enough of this macronutrient.

Every woman will have a different requirement based on her weight and her TDEE (see page 92) and for some a protein-rich mid-afternoon snack is required to avoid mindless evening snacking, which can lead to weight gain and for many becomes a habit they long to break.

Although we don't want to focus heavily on calories, it is worth noting that protein has 4 calories per gram and this goes towards your recommended daily intake.

Protein sources and amounts per 100g

	PROTEIN SOURCE	PROTEIN PER 100g	CALORIES PER 100G
Meat	chicken breast	32	128
	pork chop	31.6	127
	beef steak	31	124
	lamb chop	29.2	117
Fish	tuna (tinned in brine)	24.9	99
	salmon	20.4	82
	cod	23.9	96
	mackerel	20.3	82
	sea bass	21.5	86
	halibut	23.4	111

Seafood	sardines	19.8	80
	crab	20.5	82
	prawns	17.7	70.8
	mussels	15.4	62
	lobster	22.1	89
Eggs	boiled	14.1	57
Dairy	whole milk	3.4	130
	semi-skimmed milk	3.5	46
	skimmed milk	3.5	34
	Cheddar cheese	25.4	102
	cottage cheese	9.4	38
	plain Greek yoghurt	10	40
Pulses	fava	26.2	105
	red lentils (boiled)	7.6	31
	chickpeas (tinned)	7.2	29
Beans	tofu (steamed)	8.1	33
	black beans	6	36
	kidney beans (tinned)	6.9	28
	baked beans	5.0	20
	edamame	12	48
Grains	wheat flour	12.2	49
	rice	10.9	44
	bread (brown)	7.9	32
	bread (white)	7.9	32
	pasta	4.8	20
	porridge oats	3.0	50
Nuts and seeds	almonds	21.1	85
	walnuts	14.7	59
	hazelnuts	14.1	57
	pumpkin seeds	33	132
	chia seeds	15	60

Protein powder

Protein powder has recently come into the modern-day diet for many women on the go in order to make sure they reach their daily protein intake. However, it is really important that we don't rely solely on this source and we aim to hit those targets with food by adding protein to every meal. Protein powders contain many hidden sugars, which can play havoc with our sugar spikes, whereas protein is actually meant to play a role in controlling them.

Carbohydrates

Carbohydrates are considered to be essential nutrients by several global health organisations, including the World Health Organization, yet many of us struggle to accept that they are actually the most important source of fuel for workouts and an integral part of a healthy diet.

Many people believe that carbohydrates are the enemy of weight loss and they consider cutting out carbs or following a low-carbohydrate diet, like keto, juicing or fasting, to achieve their desired weight. There is, however, no scientific evidence that these diets are more effective than those that focus on reducing fat intake. Moreover, it's tough to stick to such diets in the long term. Low-carbohydrate diets don't allow for the healthy carbohydrates found in fruits, vegetables and whole grains, which are necessary for our bodies.

If you already have an established fitness routine or you are about to embark on this one, it is not advisable to avoid or restrict carbs as they are the main source of energy for our brains and bodies. In the meal plans that accompany the workout plan, you will see and feel how important this macronutrient is in your diet. Our bodies store carbs in our muscles as glycogen, which is then converted to glucose when we need it and is the source of energy your body requires to support bodily functions and physical activities.

Eating carbohydrates will also allow the protein to repair and rebuild muscle tissue. If we limit this, protein becomes the energy source and we will not be able to build lean muscle, meaning our workouts will not give us the results we want.

Carbohydrates have fewer calories than fat, but it is important not to consume too many. Overeating carbohydrates can lead to weight gain. The key is to consume the right type of carbohydrates in the right quantity.

It's worth noting that not all carbs are created equal. There are in fact three types of carbohydrates: sugars, starches and dietary fibre. However, these are mostly divided or dealt with in two groups, known as simple and complex carbohydrates.

Simple carbohydrates, simply put, are sugars. They are easy to digest and provide short bursts of energy. However, it's important to keep in mind that fruit, dairy and some vegetables also fall under this category and offer nutritional value.

The ones to avoid or limit would be things like fizzy drinks, sweets, chips, doughnuts, white bread, energy drinks, some cereals, fruit juices and cakes.

Complex carbohydrates take longer to digest and are the carbohydrates we want and need to eat more of. They come from whole grains and vegetables and provide a longer-lasting energy source that will keep you feeling fuller for longer.

Examples of complex 'healthy carbs' include brown rice, quinoa, sweet potatoes, potatoes, popcorn, beans, pulses, oats and wholegrain bread.

It's important to prioritise eating healthy complex carbohydrates that haven't been put through a refining process. The healthier sources of carbohydrates promote good health by delivering vitamins, minerals, fibre and a host of important phytonutrients.

Glycaemic Index (GI)

It is worth mentioning the GI index here to give an insight into how carbohydrates affect your blood sugar (glucose) levels. The GI index is a rating for food containing carbohydrates. It shows how quickly each food affects your blood sugar level (see Chapter 16) when that food is eaten on its own.

Eating foods with low GI ratings can be beneficial in managing blood glucose levels and can help control your appetite, which may be useful if you're trying to lose weight. However, it's important to keep in mind that other factors also play a role in determining blood glucose levels.

Sources of carbohydrates

Complex Carbs	Simple Carbs
High in fibre	Low in fibre
Feel full for longer	Can add to sluggish feeling
Slower release used for energy	Quick release of energy
• fruits, such as bananas, apples, grapefruit, prunes, strawberries, plums • non-starchy vegetables, spinach, carrots, tomatoes, cabbage, onions, sprouts, sweet potato, cauliflower, broccoli • whole grains, such as whole grain flour, brown rice, quinoa • peas and beans, such as black beans, lentils, peas, chickpeas • dairy and dairy products, such as low-fat milk, yoghurt	• white bread • white rice • sugar-sweetened beverages, such as sodas, fruit juices • cookies and pastries • sugary cereals • chocolate • chips • alcohol • processed foods and ready-made meals

Fats

Fat is a type of nutrient and, just like protein and carbohydrates, your body needs some fat for energy and to protect your heart and brain health. In addition, fat helps the body absorb fat-soluble vitamins, such as vitamins A, D and E.

We have been led to believe that eating fat will add inches to your waistline, raise cholesterol and cause a myriad of health problems. However, like carbohydrates, not all fat is the same.

Fats in foods can either be saturated or unsaturated. Most foods that contain fat contain a mixture of both saturated and unsaturated fats in different proportions, but we would normally describe a food as being high in saturated or unsaturated fat depending on which type they are a richer source of.

Like with carbs, by understanding the difference between good and bad fats and how to include more healthy fat in your diet, you can improve how well you think and feel, boost your energy and maintain your weight or lose weight if this is your goal.

Saturated fats

Knowing the foods that contain high amounts of saturated fat can help you make healthier choices. You do not need to eliminate saturated fat from your diet completely, but as with all these things, it's great to make informed decisions when you shop and prepare meals.

Foods that are high in saturated fats include:

- fatty cuts of meat and processed meat products like bacon, sausages and salami

- cheese, especially hard cheese like Cheddar

- cream, crème fraîche and sour cream

- butter, ghee, suet, lard

- coconut oil and palm oil

- coconut milk and cream

- ice cream

- cakes, biscuits and pastries, like pies, sausage rolls and croissants

- savoury cheese-flavoured crackers or twists

- chocolate and chocolate spreads

Unsaturated fats

Replacing saturated fats in your diet with unsaturated fats can help to maintain healthy cholesterol levels by decreasing the amount of harmful LDL cholesterol. As part of a healthy, balanced diet, choosing foods that contain higher amounts of unsaturated fat and less saturated fat can help to reduce your risk of heart disease.

There are two types of unsaturated fats: monounsaturated and polyunsaturated fats.

Monounsaturated fats

Replacing saturated fats in our diet with monounsaturated fats can help to decrease levels of total cholesterol and harmful LDL cholesterol.

Monounsaturated fats are found in:

- olive and rapeseed oils and spreads made from them

- olives

- avocados

- nuts and seeds, such as almonds, Brazil nuts, hazelnuts, peanuts, pine nuts and sesame seeds and spreads or pastes made from them (like nut butter or tahini)

These foods are typical of the Mediterranean-style diet, which is associated with good heart health and a lower risk of heart disease.

Polyunsaturated fats

Replacing saturated fats in our diet with polyunsaturated fats can also help to lower 'bad' LDL cholesterol.

There are two main types of polyunsaturated fats: omega 3 and omega 6.

Polyunsaturated fats are found in:

- some vegetable oils and spreads made from them (including corn, sunflower and sesame)

- flaxseeds, sesame seeds and sunflower seeds

- walnuts, pine nuts

- oily fish, including mackerel, salmon, trout, herring and sardines

Building a positive relationship with food

I have worked with many women who have struggled for years to have a positive relationship with food. Demonising certain food groups can lead to worrying constantly that food means weight gain, rather than seeing food as an absolute necessity to thrive and something to be enjoyed. Mostly, this is due to the fact that women aren't eating enough of the food groups I have talked about and find themselves constantly thinking about food negatively.

Over the 30 days when you are doing the plan, I would love you to follow the meals so that you can see how when you eat the right foods, in the right quantities, you can begin to change your relationship with food if this is something you have struggled with in the past.

If you have suffered or suffer from disordered eating, then please make sure you get professional help.

Calories

As we age and go through menopause, we may need to consume fewer calories. This is not the case for all women, but for those experiencing joint aches and pains who find themselves less active, this is a key component in avoiding weight gain around the middle.

As a general rule, women need to consume 1,600–2,400 calories daily to maintain their weight. Women over 60 usually need fewer calories, around 1,600–2,000 per day. However, the amount of calories you should consume depends on various factors, including age, gender, height, current weight and physical activity level.[42]

It's important to ensure you're eating enough calories to give your body the necessary nutrients, even if you're trying to lose weight. Many fad diets recommend restricting your calorie intake to around 1,000–1,200 calories per day, which is not enough for most healthy adults. Cutting your calorie intake can cause several serious side effects and also increase your risk of nutrient deficiency. Drastic eliminations will make long-term weight maintenance difficult.

Portion sizes

Using your hand as a guide effectively ensures you're consuming the right amount of food. With this simple technique, you can easily estimate serving sizes for various foods, preventing over or under-eating. Your hand is the perfect measuring tool, being proportionate to your body, consistent in size and always accessible. No need for complicated measuring or weighing.

- 1 portion of protein = 1 palm

- 1 portion of carbohydrates = 1 fist

- 1 portion of fruits and vegetables = 1 fist

- 1 portion of fat = 1 thumb

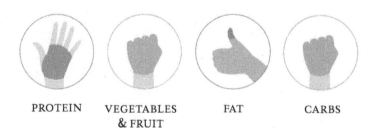

PROTEIN   VEGETABLES   FAT   CARBS
            & FRUIT

246 OWNING YOUR MENOPAUSE

Phytoestrogens

You may have heard of phytoestrogens, and you might be wondering what they are, whether they are beneficial, and how they can help. Phytoestrogens are compounds that naturally occur in plants (*phyto* is a Greek word meaning 'plant'). If you eat fruits, veggies, legumes and some grains, you get phytoestrogens from your diet. Essentially, they mimic your body's oestrogen and can alleviate some of the symptoms you are experiencing in the same way that HRT might. However, please don't see this as a replacement for HRT if you have chosen to take it.

Oestrogen, as we know, is the hormone responsible for regulating the growth, development and physiology of the human reproductive system, and is one of the essential hormones that we see declining as we go through menopause. When we eat these foods, our bodies may react as if we were producing oestrogen.

Phytoestrogens may help to prevent bone loss in ageing women. Natural oestrogen helps maintain a normal bone density, so it would make sense that if we eat a diet rich in these phytoestrogens we will be helping our bones stay strong, and potentially offsetting our risk of osteopenia and osteoporosis.[43]

Do supplements support?

It is important to ensure you are eating a balanced, nourishing diet. However, as hormones fluctuate, stress levels rise and our bodies change, it is necessary to know what and why we need certain nutrients so that we thrive from the inside out.

Katie Skrine, our in-house advisor on the Owning Your Menopause app, says, 'As a nutritionist, it is important for me to remind you that eating a balanced diet that is full of colour and variety is the best for anybody and is especially important during menopause.'

Katie has provided us with a guide to the key nutrients we need, how we can find them and the role they play in supporting us through this transition.

Key nutrients and where to find them

Nutrient	Where can I find it?	Why do I need it?
C (ascorbic acid)	Red peppers, oranges, kiwis, mango, berries, tomatoes, broccoli, green leafy vegetables, parsley, blackcurrants and frozen peas Eat every day	Vitamin C is a powerful antioxidant and easy to consume. It improves the health of our cells, heart and immune system and can help at times of stress – a common symptom of perimenopause. It also helps to produce collagen, which is in decline at this stage of our life.
B6	Milk, salmon, tuna, eggs, chicken liver, beef, carrots, spinach, sweet potato, green peas, bananas, chickpeas, cereal and avocado Incorporate these into your diet daily	Curtails low mood, mood swings and depression by helping to produce a key chemical messenger, serotonin. During menopause, serotonin levels fluctuate or drop, which can also contribute to brain fog, dizziness, heart palpitations, vertigo and memory problems.
B12	Most commonly found in animal products – fish, meat, poultry and eggs	Key for boosting energy, brain health, memory, bone health and your overall mood and well-being. If you are vegetarian and suffer from low energy, fatigue, memory loss, constipation, loss of appetite, numbness and tingling in the hands and feet or depression, it would be well worth getting your B12 levels tested with your GP.
Calcium	Dairy or fortified plant milk, fish with bones (tinned sardines and whitebait), tofu, spinach, broccoli, white beans, dried figs, almonds, oranges, kale and watercress Under the age of 50, women need around 700mg a day of calcium, but post-50 this increases to 1200mg per day	Calcium depletes with age and especially in women after menopause. It is essential for healthy bones, teeth, heart and muscles. Unless advised by your doctor, stay away from supplementing.

Vitamin D	Expose your skin to sunshine! Other sources are fatty fish, fish liver oils, beef liver, cheese, egg yolks and fortified foods. Include in your daily diet as much as you can and get outside in the sunshine daily	Vitamin D is important for bone health to help prevent brittle bones or bone pain, and osteomalacia (softening of the bones). It is also important for a healthy immune system. Although you can get from a few food sources, the sun is your best source. It is, for this reason, a nutrient we do need to supplement, especially in the West and during the winter.
Folate (B9)	Dark green leafy vegetables, beans, peanuts, sunflower seeds, fresh fruits and whole grains	Folic acid, or folate, is needed to form DNA and plays an important role in breaking down protein and producing healthy red blood cells. Signs of low levels include anaemia, weight loss, weakness, head-aches and it is a risk factor for heart disease. Folic acid can also help reduce hot flushes.
Omega 3	Oily fish – SMASH: sardines, mackerel, anchovies, salmon, herrings – tinned, fresh or frozen. Aim for 2–3 palm-size servings per week	A long-chain fatty acid that your body can't produce, so you must include it in your diet. Crucial for every cell in your body, as well as being anti-inflammatory and key for brain health. If you don't eat fish, it may be worth looking into a good supplement. Make sure it contains the two most impor-tant types of omega 3: EPA and DHA.
Magnesium	Almonds, green leafy vegeta-bles, black beans, avocado, pumpkin seeds, whole grains and dark chocolate In addition, add Epsom salts to your evening bath and soak for 20 minutes to help absorb the salts	Magnesium is an important mineral and it can help improve mood, promote healthy bones and hormone levels and is important for our energy production, as well as for improving sleep.

CHAPTER 19

Limit or Avoid

Throughout this book, I have highlighted the importance of adding weights to your workouts and looked at how many other external factors can have a huge influence on your symptoms.

Movement and implementing a balanced, nourishing diet, plus HRT for those who can and choose to use it, will see you make some positive steps towards a stronger you, however, there are a few more considerations to factor in if you are still struggling.

I work with many women who, despite having made these changes and feeling so much better, would like to make more progress. When I sit down and talk to them, I often find out that some of the foods and drinks they are consuming are playing a role and are hindering them from making this happen.

I never want women to think that they have to make sacrifices on their quest to feeling strong in mind and body as they navigate menopause, and I hate demonising foods or drinks, but I repeatedly see how the effects of alcohol and caffeine can stop many women from allowing themselves the best opportunity to thrive at this time.

I have worked with and seen so many women remove alcohol from their lives and make incredible progress really quickly. To this end, I will be encouraging you to do the 30-Day Plan alongside a period of sobriety.

While coffee isn't as much of a hindrance as alcohol, it can exacerbate many symptoms and play havoc with your sleep patterns.

Caffeine

To help manage hot flushes, limit your intake of caffeinated drinks, such as coffee and tea, or choose decaffeinated versions and herbal infusions instead. It is best to avoid drinking caffeinated beverages close to bedtime as this may also contribute to poor sleep.

Sugar

Sugar can add to your stress because high glucose levels (see Chapter 16) can increase your cortisol. An increase in cortisol affects the amount of progesterone you make, which can exacerbate menopausal symptoms alongside your already fluctuating hormones. Signs of this include heavier bleeding and more irregularities with your cycle, and it can also negatively impact anxiety, mood, sweats and hot flushes.

Not only this, but sugar has a significant impact on oestrogen. The fluctuating and declining levels may reduce your insulin sensitivity, meaning you cannot clear sugar as efficiently from the blood. This puts you at a greater risk of Type 2 diabetes, weight gain and low mood.

Naturally declining oestrogen can also impact the functionality of your thyroid, which plays a crucial role in setting your metabolic rate and energy production. As a result, you may experience higher levels of fatigue. Unfortunately, this low energy may lead to an increased desire for more sugar-rich foods as a pick-me-up, creating a vicious cycle of dependence on sugar.

In Chapter 17, we talked about our gut health and the microbiome, which is crucial to our overall well-being. As Katie Skrine explained, a diet high in sugar feeds non-beneficial bacteria and leads to the colonisation of harmful yeasts and bacteria. This can result in uncomfortable issues like bloating, digestive upset and an increased risk of conditions like urinary tract infections (UTIs) and thrush. Women going through menopause can experience vaginal atrophy (see Chapter 2) and be more susceptible to UTIs, making it even more important to watch your sugar intake.

Alcohol

Mood swings, sleepless nights, feelings of insecurity and anxiety are some of the symptoms you may experience as you head through menopause. The experience can be so stressful that who could blame any of us for wanting to decompress with a glass of wine or two?

The reality, however, is that drinking worsens mood swings, sleepless nights, insecurities and anxiety. I talk a lot about lifestyle changes to improve your menopause symptoms. Putting exercise aside, my number one must-change is, without a doubt, cutting back or quitting alcohol.

In terms of the 30-Day Plan, disrupted sleep from alcohol can lead to slow muscle gain because interrupted sleep patterns can hinder muscle growth. That means all that excellent movement you are doing is being single-handedly counteracted by drinking too much alcohol.

Not only that, but we know that alcohol dehydrates. Dehydration also leads to reduced exercise performance. You need to be well-hydrated when you exercise to maintain blood flow through your body, which carries oxygen and nutrients to your muscles, maximising performance and, more importantly, avoiding injury.

Women are less alcohol-tolerant than men are.[44] This is partly because our bodies tend to be smaller. We also have less alcohol dehydrogenase, an enzyme that metabolises alcohol in the stomach.[45] Plus, that enzyme is relatively inactive in the liver of women. As a result, we tend to absorb far more alcohol into our bloodstream than men. Meanwhile, as we age, our bodies lose water volume. As a result, we are less able to dilute any alcohol in our systems. That makes us that much more vulnerable to its effects.[46]

We know that alcohol can be more dangerous the older you get, especially for women, but what I find really worrying is that the prevalence of binge drinking is rising among women navigating menopause. Heavy drinking is associated with the following health risks:

- all cancers, especially breast cancer

- heart disease

- osteoporosis / bone mass loss

- depression

- sleep disruption

- memory loss

- can put organs at risk of damage

- increased blood pressure

Drinking alcohol also adds unnecessary stress on your adrenal glands, and therefore increases the stress hormone cortisol (see Chapter 16), which often means that after the initial high leaves, what seemed like fun at the time can have the opposite effect, leaving you feeling low and tired. This can show up as depression for some.

Having an understanding of what it is your body needs to fuel, rebuild and nourish itself is key to your success. Without good nutrition, you will find that any fitness progress you want to make will be slow. The two go hand-in-hand and once you experience how good you can feel and how you have the opportunity to thrive at this time, making these small adjustments and tweaks will become much easier and more sustainable.

> *My takeaways from the plan are that I don't miss alcohol. I had a drink every night as a crutch for perimenopause symptoms. I had reduced it to a few nights a week before discovering the OYM plan, but I know that was still too much. I don't think I'll ever go back to drinking as often. Thank you for that. I have realised eating healthily doesn't have to be a lot of work. I also had sweet cravings and often felt an afternoon slump. That's sorted now thanks to extra protein in my meals and liquorice tea.*
>
> **Katie**

You want to make the way in which you eat and nourish your body something that you can see yourself sticking to. It's time to hop off the hamster wheel of diets and implement changes that you can stick to 365 days a year. If you start making the changes today, the benefits you feel will motivate you to stick at it.

Summary

- Protein is an absolute non-negotiable and you must try to add it to every meal. Protein is essential in order to help you feel fuller for longer and for your body to repair and build lean muscle.

- Reduce or cut out alcohol completely as this will exacerbate many of the symptoms you may be experiencing.

- Less is not more when it comes to nourishing and fuelling your menopausal body. Aiming for THREE balanced meals a day with a gap of 4–5 hours in between can make huge difference.

- Your digestive health is essential for your body to carry out many day-to-day functions and having a varied diet rich in fibre and making sure you have a colourful plate is key to supporting your gut microbiome. Having good gut bacteria can help your body's immune system and alleviate many of the symptoms associated with menopause.

PART 6

Menus, Recipes and Meal Plans

This is where you will find a collection of nourishing, fuelling and delicious meals to accompany the 30-Day Plan. These meals will ensure you are consuming and hitting targets on all the food groups we have talked about.

When you are navigating menopause and working out, eating this way will make a huge difference in making you feel fitter, calmer and stronger. It will keep you feeling full, help boost energy levels and may even improve your sleep if this is something you have been struggling with.

It will also help with recovery and repair after you embark on this new regime and your mind and body will reward you and thank you.

Please note that you don't have to follow the plan meal by meal. The key to success is understanding the basic principles of healthy eating, prioritising fuelling your body so it can thrive and getting into the habit of planning so there are always healthy meal options available.

Some people like a structure to follow as they develop new habits, so I have made it easy with these plans and lists. However, you may well be pretty familiar with some of these strategies, so it's completely fine to adapt the meals to fit around your lifestyle, work pattern and family responsibilities.

So, I haven't stuck to the plan 100 per cent but I am so far better than I was 21 days ago.

I'm much more aware of getting a variety of plants in my diet and am having a lot more than I was previously and ensuring I have protein at every meal. I'm more in tune with when I feel hungry and not and don't eat at a specific time for the sake of it.

Even after this short time I'm feeling stronger, which is great.

Yes, I still have room for improvement but this a great start and unlike other things I've tried, I feel that I can keep up the changes and keep on working on the other stuff I would like to improve.

Alix

To achieve progress and change, I encourage you to follow these principles

- Don't get caught up in calorie counting. We all have different portion requirements, and it's best to learn and understand what you need intuitively. I have included it in the recipes for guidance purposes only.

- Notice how the food makes you feel – write it down.

- If you are full, don't feel obligated to finish the entire meal.

- Allow time between meals, approximately 4–5 hours. This plan isn't about picking at food; instead, it's about eating substantial meals to keep yourself full and avoid snacking mindlessly.

- Don't skip meals.

- Try to avoid gulping water before, during and after meals.

- Drink 2 litres of water throughout the day and unlimited herbal tea.

- Avoid alcohol (if you really can't, then 1–2 glasses a week MAX).

- Limit caffeine after midday.

- Try to walk for 10 minutes after your lunch.

- Plan and prepare for the week ahead.

Suggested daily timings for meals

- Breakfast 9 am

- Lunch 1.30 pm

- Supper 7 pm

This plan is designed to help you achieve balance, enjoy your meals and make small changes that can have a significant impact on your health.

For those busy days when you're on the go, I've included three quick-and-easy options perfect for breakfasts and lunch at your desk or while you're out and about. Having three meals a day will help you to get the most out of the plan, so please don't skip meals.

The meal plan and exercise plan aim to:

- help alleviate symptoms

- encourage you to see how little change can make a big difference

- boost energy and well-being

- help you prioritise you and your nutrition

Don't let the abundance of information on perimenopause and menopause overwhelm or confuse you. Keep it simple by focusing on implementing small, sustainable changes over 30 days. This way, you can discover which foods support your body during this time, form healthier habits and relish every meal. Remember, your success depends on making realistic and sustainable changes that will last a lifetime.

Self sabotage

Much of sticking to a plan is about balance but as we have said, it is also about making it fun so you can stick with it. If you go out one night and make choices that might not be the best, that's OK. Don't be tempted to hit the 'sod it' button.

We convince ourselves that it has all gone to pot, and then we think we're back to square one. That couldn't be further from the truth. In those situations, what I would love to encourage you to do is just to stop and recognise what you've done is OK. Have fun. Park it.

As long as this only happens occasionally, it won't affect the progress you are making. Enjoy that moment rather than feeling guilty about it. Move on to the next day and return to making those sensible food choices you set yourself for the rest of the week.

Please note

If you are a vegetarian or vegan, I have tried to give alternatives. You can use leftovers the next day for lunch or dinner.

Planning, prepping and batch cooking

One of the key ways to ensure you succeed is to plan your week ahead and see where you can try to batch cook. I know how time-poor many of us are, but what I would like you to see is that with a bit of forward planning you can eat three delicious meals a day, without always defaulting to a salad.

Many of the dishes included here can be made in advance, which will help you manage your time.

I love the flexibility of the exercise and meal plan. I'm fitting it in well with cooking for my family. I have young kids and I think I can sustain what I am currently doing. I am thinking twice about snacking or what I am considering eating with nutritive value in mind.

Lindsay

THE FITTER, CALMER, STRONGER IN 30 DAYS MEAL PLAN

	DAY 1	DAY 2	DAY 3	DAY 4	DAY 5	DAY 6	DAY 7
Breakfast	Overnight Oats	Chia Seed Pot	Chia Seed Pot	Blueberry Protein Pancakes	Simple Protein Pancakes	Spinach Shakshuka	Healthy Granola
Lunch	Grilled Chicken or Tofu & Pineapple Salad	Sweet Potato, Quinoa & Bean Burgers	Tuna or Tofu & Quinoa Toss Salad	Grilled Chicken or Tofu & Pineapple Salad	Tuna or Tofu & Quinoa Toss Salad	Sweet Potato, Quinoa & Bean Burgers	**Roast of choice** or Quinoa & Beetroot Salad
Dinner	Creamy Chicken, Mushroom & Spinach Pasta	Miso Salmon or Tofu with Courgetti Noodles	Creamy Chicken, Mushroom & Spinach Pasta	Curried Cauli-flower Soup	Chicken Thighs with Hoisin Rice	Fish Curry	**Roast of choice** or Quinoa & Beetroot Salad

	DAY 8	DAY 9	DAY 10	DAY 11	DAY 12	DAY 13	DAY 14
Breakfast	Healthy Granola	Straw-berry Protein Bowl	Chia Seed Pot	Chia Seed Pot	Simple Protein Pancakes	Chickpea Scramble	Blueberry Protein Pancakes
Lunch	Curried Cauli-flower Soup	Quinoa & Beetroot Salad	Curried Cauli-flower Soup	Wild Rice, Tomato & Rocket Balsamic Salad	Sweet Potato Curry	Potato Pancakes with Cottage Cheese	**Roast of choice** or Quinoa & Beetroot Salad
Dinner	Prosciutto-wrapped Chicken with Lentils	Tofu or Salmon Pad Thai	Sweet Potato Curry	Creamy Chicken, Mushroom & Tomato Pasta	Miso Salmon or Tofu with Courgetti Noodles	Chicken Thighs with Hoisin Rice	**Roast of choice** or Curried Cauli-flower Soup

	DAY 15	DAY 16	DAY 17	DAY 18	DAY 19	DAY 20	DAY 21
Breakfast	Overnight Oats	Chia Seed Pot	Chia Seed Pot	Blueberry Protein Pancakes	Simple Protein Pancakes	Spinach Shakshuka	Healthy Granola
Lunch	Grilled Chicken or Tofu & Pineapple Salad	Sweet Potato, Quinoa & Bean Burgers	Tuna or Tofu & Quinoa Toss Salad	Grilled Chicken or Tofu & Pineapple Salad	Tuna or Tofu & Quinoa Toss Salad	Sweet Potato, Quinoa & Bean Burgers	**Roast of choice** or Quinoa & Beetroot Salad
Dinner	Creamy Chicken, Mushroom & Spinach Pasta	Miso Salmon or Tofu with Courgetti Noodles	Creamy Chicken, Mushroom & Tomato Pasta	Curried Cauli-flower Soup	Chicken Thighs with Hoisin Rice	Fish Curry	**Roast of choice** or Quinoa & Beetroot Salad

	DAY 22	DAY 23	DAY 24	DAY 25	DAY 26	DAY 27	DAY 28
Breakfast	Healthy Granola	Straw-berry Protein Bowl	Chia Seed Pot	Chia Seed Pot	Simple Protein Pancakes	Chickpea Scramble	Blueberry Protein Pancakes
Lunch	Curried Cauli-flower Soup	Quinoa & Beetroot Salad	Curried Cauli-flower Soup	Wild Rice, Tomato & Rocket Balsamic Salad	Sweet Potato Curry	Potato Pancakes with Cottage Cheese	**Roast of choice** or Quinoa & Beetroot Salad
Dinner	Prosciutto-wrapped Chicken with Lentils	Tofu or Salmon Pad Thai	Sweet Potato Curry	Creamy Chicken, Mushroom & Tomato Pasta	Miso Salmon or Tofu with Courgetti Noodles	Chicken Thighs with Hoisin Rice	**Roast of choice** or Curried Cauli-flower Soup

	DAY 29	DAY 30
Breakfast	Chickpea Scramble	Blueberry Protein Pancakes
Lunch	Curried Cauli-flower Soup	Quinoa & Beetroot Salad
Dinner	Creamy Chicken, Mushroom & Spinach Pasta	Prosciutto-wrapped Chicken with Lentils

Breakfasts

Simple Protein Pancakes (Serves 4)

80g oats

5 eggs

225g cottage cheese

2 tsp ground cinnamon

1 tbsp maple syrup

2 tsp coconut oil, for frying

1 banana, sliced

30g walnuts, chopped

- Place the oats, eggs, cottage cheese, ground cinnamon and maple syrup in a food processor or blender and blend.
- Heat a medium frying pan over a low heat and add ½ teaspoon of the coconut oil.
- Add a quarter of the pancake batter to form a small pancake.
- Cook until golden brown. Repeat with the remaining mix.
- Top with the sliced banana and walnuts. Serve immediately.

Note: Add another 50g Greek yoghurt for more protein.

Prep	Cook	Kcal	Fats(g)	Carbs(g)	Protein(g)
5 mins	15 mins	298	17	20	17

Chia Seed Pot (Serves 1)

2 tbsp chia seeds

125ml oat milk, or substitute for any plant milk/milk

2 tsp maple syrup, plus a drizzle to serve

fruit, such as berries, banana, kiwis or mango, to serve

- Combine the chia seeds, milk and maple syrup in a jar or bowl.
- Cover and chill overnight or for at least 3 hours.

- When ready to serve, top with fruit and a drizzle of maple syrup.

Prep	Chill	Kcal	Fats(g)	Carbs(g)	Protein(g)
5 mins	3 hours	230	11	21	5

Blueberry Protein Pancakes (Serves 1)

3 eggs

25g ground almonds

½ banana, mashed

25g frozen blueberries

plant milk/milk

½ tsp coconut oil

- Whisk together the eggs and ground almonds.
- Stir in the mashed banana and add the blueberries. If the pancake mixture seems too thick, add a splash of your chosen milk to thin it.
- Heat the coconut oil in a medium frying pan over a low-medium heat. Pour in the pancake mixture to make three small pancakes and cook until little bubbles form, about 5 minutes.
- Make sure the pancakes have set enough before flipping them over. Cook the pancakes for another 2–3 minutes.

Prep	Cook	Kcal	Fats(g)	Carbs(g)	Protein(g)
5 mins	10 mins	257	5	18	36

Strawberry Protein Bowl (Serves 4)

600g cottage cheese

225g frozen strawberries,
   thawed

4 tbsp maple syrup

170g healthy granola (see
   below or shop-bought)

150g fresh berries

Optional toppings

walnuts

sunflower seeds

pumpkin seeds

- Place the cottage cheese, strawberries and maple syrup in a food processor or high-speed blender and blitz until smooth and creamy.
- Divide among four serving bowls and top with granola, fresh berries and your choice of optional toppings, to serve.

Prep	Cook	Kcal	Fats(g)	Carbs(g)	Protein(g)
15 mins	0 mins	315	10	37	19

Healthy Granola (Serves 16)

160g rolled oats

115g walnuts, chopped

1 tbsp ground cinnamon

pinch of salt

4 tbsp almond butter

120ml maple syrup

- Preheat the oven to 160°C (325°F) and line a baking tray with baking paper.
- Mix the oats, walnuts and cinnamon in a large bowl, adding a pinch of salt.
- Next, add the almond butter and maple syrup and mix until well combined and sticky.
- Spread the mixture evenly over the baking tray and bake for 15 minutes on the middle shelf in the oven. Remove the tray, stir the mixture to break it up a little, and place back

in the oven to cook for a further 10–12 minutes until golden brown.
- Remove the tray from the oven and place on a wire rack to cool. Once cooled down, store in an airtight container for up to a week.

Note: Top with Greek yoghurt for added protein.

Prep	Cook	Kcal	Fats(g)	Carbs(g)	Protein(g)
10 mins	30 mins	166	8.2	16.8	8

Spinach Shakshuka (Serves 2)

1 tbsp coconut oil
1 large onion, chopped
2 garlic cloves, crushed
300g mushrooms, sliced

450g spinach
4 eggs
handful of parsley, chopped

- Heat the oil in a large pan over a medium heat. Add the onion and garlic and cook for 2–3 minutes until soft. Next, add the mushrooms and cook for another 3–4 minutes. Season with salt and pepper.
- Now start adding the spinach to the pan – you will likely have to do this in batches. Cover the pan with a lid and let it wilt. Repeat this step until all the spinach is in the pan. Stir well and taste for seasoning.
- Make four indentations ('wells') in the spinach and break an egg into each. Cook for 5–6 minutes, covered with a lid, until the egg whites are set.
- Scatter with chopped parsley and serve.

Prep	Cook	Kcal	Fats(g)	Carbs(g)	Protein(g)
10 mins	15 mins	321	22	19	24

Chickpea Scramble (Serves 2)

330g tinned chickpeas,
   rinsed and drained
½ tsp turmeric
½ tsp paprika
2 tsp olive oil

1 small onion, finely diced
2 garlic cloves, finely
   chopped
230g spinach
½ avocado

- Mash the chickpeas with a fork, leaving some whole. Mix in the turmeric and paprika and season with salt and pepper.
- Heat the oil in a medium frying pan over a medium-high heat and sauté the onion and garlic for 2–3 minutes until fragrant.
- Add the mashed chickpeas and cook for another 5 minutes, then transfer to a bowl, cover with foil and set aside. Using the same pan, wilt the spinach, adding a tablespoon of water.
- Once ready, divide the spinach between two bowls, top with the chickpeas and serve each with ¼ avocado.

Prep	Cook	Kcal	Fats(g)	Carbs(g)	Protein(g)
10 mins	15 mins	417	15	56	19

On-the-go options

Breakfast Oat Cookies (Makes 9)

90g rolled oats
30g ground almonds
3 tbsp desiccated coconut
1 tsp ground cinnamon
¼ tsp bicarbonate of soda
3 tbsp almond butter

3 tbsp maple syrup
1 medium ripe banana,
   mashed
handful of fresh berries

- Preheat the oven to 160°C (325°F) and line a baking tray with baking paper.
- Place all the ingredients (apart from the berries) in a medium bowl and mix well, then place the mixture in the freezer for 10–15 minutes.
- Using slightly wet hands, create nine balls out of the mixture and place them on the baking tray, pushing them down to create cookie shapes. Gently press a few berries onto each cookie.
- Bake for 20 minutes until golden. Allow to cool completely before eating.

Note: The cookies will keep for up to 2–3 days in a sealed container.

Prep	Cook	Kcal	Fats(g)	Carbs(g)	Protein(g)
10 mins	20 mins	137	6	17	3

Protein Smoothie (Serves 1)

240ml almond milk
150g frozen berries
1 banana

1 medium beetroot, cooked
and grated
25g vanilla protein powder

- Add all the ingredients into a blender. Pulse until smooth, then pour into a glass and serve immediately or bottle it up ready to enjoy later.

Prep	Cook	Kcal	Fats(g)	Carbs(g)	Protein(g)
5 mins	0 mins	230	6.8	32	12

Overnight Oats (Serves 1)

· ·

40g oats
100ml plant milk/milk
50g Greek yoghurt

Optional toppings
blueberries
banana
strawberries

- Place the oats in a Tupperware or similar type of container.
- Add the milk and yoghurt and stir. The milk should just cover the oats.
- Cover and leave in the fridge overnight.
- Add toppings before heading out or serving.

Prep	Cook	Kcal	Fats(g)	Carbs(g)	Protein(g)
5 mins	0 mins	381	12	37	15

Lunches

Curried Cauliflower Soup (Serves 2)

· ·

1 cauliflower	1 onion, chopped
2 tbsp olive oil	190g dried red lentils
2 tsp fennel seeds	3 tbsp yellow curry paste

- Preheat the oven to 200°C (400°F).
- Separate the cauliflower head into small florets.
- Drizzle a quarter of the cauliflower with 1 tablespoon of olive oil and season with 1 teaspoon of the fennel seeds and some salt and pepper.
- Place in a roasting dish and set aside.
- Heat the remaining 1 tablespoon of oil in a large pan, adding the chopped onion and the remaining 1 teaspoon of fennel seeds.
- Cook for 3–4 minutes until the onion has softened.
- Add the remaining cauliflower and lentils to the pan.
- Stir in the curry paste and add 1 litre of water.
- Bring to a boil, then reduce the heat and simmer gently for 25 minutes until the cauliflower is tender and the lentils are cooked.
- In the meantime, place the roasting dish with the cauliflower into the oven and roast for 20 minutes, until browned.
- Once the soup is cooked, blitz it with a hand blender until smooth and creamy.
- To serve, divide the soup into bowls and top with the roasted cauliflower.

Prep	Cook	Kcal	Fats(g)	Carbs(g)	Protein(g)
10 mins	30 mins	296	8	44	15

Brown Rice, Tomato & Rocket Balsamic Salad (Serves 4)

185g brown rice
160g roasted peppers,
  drained and chopped
30g roasted almonds,
  chopped

150g cherry tomatoes,
  halved
60g rocket
1 tbsp balsamic vinegar
1 tbsp olive oil
½ tsp chilli flakes

- Cook the rice according to the instructions on the packet. Once cooked, place in a large bowl.
- Add the peppers, almonds, tomatoes and rocket, then drizzle with vinegar and oil and add the chilli flakes. Season to taste with salt and pepper and mix well before serving.

Prep	Cook	Kcal	Fats(g)	Carbs(g)	Protein(g)
10 mins	20 mins	288	9	44	7

Sweet Potato Curry (Serves 4)

2 tsp coconut oil
1 onion, diced
2 garlic cloves, finely
   chopped
4 tbsp Thai red curry paste
2 sweet potatoes, peeled and
   diced
400g tin chopped tomatoes
240ml vegetable stock
65g smooth natural peanut

butter
120ml tinned coconut milk
juice of 1 lime

To serve
2 x 250g packets cooked
   brown rice
30g peanuts, chopped
handful of coriander,
   chopped

- Melt the coconut oil in a large pan over a medium heat. Add the onion and cook for about 5 minutes until soft.
- Next, add the garlic and red curry paste and stir well. Add the sweet potato, chopped tomatoes and vegetable stock and season with salt and pepper. Bring to a boil, then reduce the heat to medium-low and simmer for 30–35 minutes until the sweet potato is tender.
- In a small bowl, whisk together the peanut butter and coconut milk. Pour into the pan and stir well to combine.
- Remove from the heat, squeeze in the lime juice, mix well and serve with the hot rice. Garnish with the chopped peanuts and coriander.

Prep	Cook	Kcal	Fats(g)	Carbs(g)	Protein(g)
10 mins	40 mins	459	18	62	13

Potato Pancakes with Cottage Cheese (Serves 1)

140g potatoes, peeled and finely grated
50g courgette, finely grated
1 egg
½ shallot, chopped
2 tbsp chopped dill
2 tbsp spelt flour

Topping
2 radishes, finely chopped
½ shallot, finely chopped
1 tbsp chopped dill
50g cottage cheese
1 tbsp Greek yoghurt

- Place the potato and courgette in a bowl and add the egg, shallot, dill, flour and salt and pepper. Mix well until combined to make the pancake batter.
- Heat up a non-stick frying pan and fry small pancakes for 3 minutes, then flip and fry for another 1 minute.
- Mix the chopped radish and shallot with the dill, cheese and yoghurt. Season to taste with salt and pepper.
- Serve the pancakes warm with the cheese mix on top.

Prep	Cook	Kcal	Fats(g)	Carbs(g)	Protein(g)
10 mins	5 mins	502	20	56	28

Quinoa & Beetroot Salad (Serves 4)

2 x 250g packets cooked
  quinoa
200g feta cheese, cubed
2 medium beetroots, cooked
  and cubed

165g tinned chickpeas, rinsed
  and drained
2 tbsp olive oil
finely grated zest and juice of
  1 lemon

- Combine the cooked quinoa, feta cheese, beetroot and chick-peas in a medium-sized bowl. Drizzle with olive oil and lemon juice and add the lemon zest.
- Season to taste with salt and pepper and mix well to combine. Divide among four plates and serve immediately.

Prep	Cook	Kcal	Fats(g)	Carbs(g)	Protein(g)
10 mins	0 mins	395	21	38	16

Grilled Chicken or Tofu & Pineapple Salad (Serves 2)

Dressing
2 tbsp olive oil
1 tsp grated ginger
1 garlic clove, finely chopped
juice of 1 lime
1 tsp honey
Tabasco (optional)

Salad
2 handfuls of salad leaves or
  spinach
10g mint leaves
200g chicken breast or tofu
4 slices of tinned pineapple
½ small onion, finely chopped

- Mix the ingredients for the dressing in a salad bowl and season with salt. Add the spinach or salad leaves and mint leaves and let it rest.
- In the meantime, cut the chicken breasts in half, horizontally (you will end up with four chicken fillets), place in a hot grill pan, cover each chicken piece with a slice of pineapple and

season with black pepper. Grill for around 6–8 minutes, then turn and grill for another 5 minutes (at this stage, remove the pineapple and let it grill next to the chicken).

- If using tofu, cut into slices and place on a hot grill pan. Grill for around 4 minutes, then turn and grill for another 4 minutes. Grill the pineapple slices next to the tofu.
- Remove from the heat and let the chicken or tofu rest for 3 minutes, then cut it into strips.
- Add the chicken or tofu to the salad together with the pineapple and finely chopped onion, mixing before serving.

Prep	Cook	Kcal	Fats(g)	Carbs(g)	Protein(g)
10 mins	15 mins	356	16	34	27 chicken 15 tofu

Tuna or Tofu & Quinoa Toss Salad (Serves 2)

Dressing
1 tbsp olive oil
2 tsp red wine vinegar
1 tsp fresh lemon juice
1 tsp Dijon mustard

Salad
2 x 250g packets cooked
    quinoa

50g tinned chickpeas, rinsed
    and drained
½ cucumber, chopped
1 tbsp crumbled feta cheese
10 cherry tomatoes, halved
2 tins tuna (200g drained) or
    200g tofu

- Combine the dressing ingredients in a small bowl, then combine the cooked quinoa and the other salad ingredients in a separate bowl. If using tofu, cube and gently fry until golden brown, about 5–7 minutes.
- Drizzle the salad with the dressing and toss gently to coat.

Prep	Cook (tofu)	Kcal	Fats(g)	Carbs(g)	Protein(g)
10 mins	10 mins	399	11	41	37

Sweet Potato, Quinoa & Bean Burgers (Serves 4)

• •

1 sweet potato
1½ tbsp olive oil
1 tsp chopped rosemary
½ tsp chilli flakes
60g raw quinoa

400g tin kidney beans, rinsed
   and drained
25g salad leaves
25g Greek yoghurt

- Preheat the oven to 210°C (410°F) and cut the sweet potato into 2cm pieces. Place in an ovenproof dish, drizzle with ½ tablespoon of the olive oil and season with salt and pepper, rosemary and chilli flakes. Roast for 25–30 minutes.
- Meanwhile, cook the quinoa according to the instructions on the packet.
- Once the potatoes are cooked, allow them to cool slightly, then peel off the skins, place the flesh in a bowl and mash with a fork. Add the drained beans and also mash with a fork.
- Once the quinoa is cooked, transfer to the mashed beans and potato, season with salt and pepper and mix well.
- Using slightly wet hands, form four burgers and grease each one with the remaining olive oil. Place on a baking tray lined with foil and bake for 20–25 minutes.
- Serve the burgers on a bed of leaves with a dollop of Greek yoghurt for added protein.

Prep	Cook	Kcal	Fats(g)	Carbs(g)	Protein(g)
10 mins	55 mins	171	6	22	10

Dinners

Tofu or Salmon Pad Thai (Serves 2)

. . . .

Sauce
60ml tamari or soy sauce
60ml maple syrup
3 tbsp water
2 tbsp rice vinegar
2 tbsp peanut butter
1 tbsp sriracha

Tofu or salmon
200g firm tofu, pressed (see Note) and cubed or salmon fillet
1 tbsp flour
1 tbsp coconut oil

Pad Thai
225g thick rice noodles
1 tbsp coconut oil
2 shallots, chopped
2 large carrots, sliced into ribbons or matchsticks
3 garlic cloves, finely chopped
2 handfuls of bean sprouts
3 spring onions, sliced (green part)
30g peanuts, chopped
1 lime, cut into wedges

- Mix all the sauce ingredients in a bowl and set aside.
- In a large bowl, toss the tofu (if using) with flour and season with salt, making sure all the sides are coated, then set aside.
- Cook the noodles according to the instructions on the packet.
- If using tofu, heat the coconut oil in a wok or large frying pan over a medium-high heat. Add the prepared tofu cubes and cook for 1–2 minutes until brown. Remove from the heat and set aside.
- If using salmon, heat the coconut oil in a wok or large frying pan over a medium-high heat. Turn the heat down, add the salmon and cook for 7–10 minutes, turning once. Remove from the pan and set aside.
- Now, add the oil for the pad Thai to the wok and heat. Add the shallot, carrot and garlic and stir-fry for 1–2 minutes until

softened, then add in the earlier prepared sauce and noodles and cook for 1 minute.

- Next, add the tofu or salmon and bean sprouts and gently mix until well combined.
- Remove from the heat and top with the green part of the spring onions. Serve with peanuts and lime wedges.

Note: To press the tofu, wrap a block of tofu in a few paper towels and place it on a plate. Place a cast-iron frying pan on top (or something heavy) and let it drain for about 15 minutes or more. Pat dry to remove excess moisture on the surface.

Prep	Cook	Kcal	Fats(g)	Carbs(g)	Protein(g)
15 mins	15 mins	469	18	68	15

Chicken Thighs with Hoisin Rice (Serves 4)

. . . .

2 tbsp coconut oil

8 skinless chicken thighs

4 garlic cloves, sliced

4 spring onions, chopped

200g jasmine rice

200ml white wine

500ml hot chicken stock

4 tbsp dried cranberries

Hoisin sauce

3 tbsp soy sauce

2 tbsp rice vinegar

1 tbsp peanut butter

1 tsp chilli flakes

1 tsp honey

1 tsp sesame oil

- Preheat the oven to 190°C (375°F).
- In a large pan, heat the coconut oil.
- Season the chicken thighs with salt and pepper and fry for 5 minutes on each side until golden brown, then remove from the heat and transfer to a plate.
- Pour out most of the fat from the pan, leaving about 1 tablespoon.
- Add into the pan the sliced garlic and the spring onions. Sauté for 1 minute.
- Add the uncooked rice and fry again for about 1 minute. Pour in the wine and cook for a further 2 minutes until most of the liquid evaporates. Next, add the hot stock and cranberries and all the ingredients for the hoisin sauce. Bring to a boil.
- Transfer the rice to an ovenproof dish and place the chicken thighs in the centre. Bake for 30 minutes.
- Once cooked, divide among plates and serve, or store in the fridge for up to 2–3 days.

Prep	Cook	Kcal	Fats(g)	Carbs(g)	Protein(g)
5 mins	50 mins	336	15	16	29

Prosciutto-wrapped Chicken with Lentils (Serves 2)

. . . .

4 skinless chicken thighs (about 480g)

8 tsp red pesto

8 prosciutto slices

2 x 400g tins lentils, rinsed and drained

145g sun-dried tomatoes, drained

2 tbsp apple cider vinegar

2 tbsp oil, from the sun-dried tomatoes

- Preheat the oven to 180°C (350°F).
- Cut each chicken thigh into two pieces and season with salt and pepper. Spread 1 teaspoon of pesto over each piece of chicken and wrap in a slice of prosciutto. Place on a baking tray and bake for 25–30 minutes until crispy and cooked through.
- In the meantime, place the lentils and tomatoes in a pan and gently warm them through, adding the apple cider vinegar and 2 tablespoons of oil from the sun-dried tomatoes.
- Divide the lentils among four plates and top with the chicken. Serve immediately.

Prep	Cook	Kcal	Fats(g)	Carbs(g)	Protein(g)
15 mins	30 mins	462	14	41	46

Fish Curry (Serves 4)

. . . .

1 tbsp olive oil
1 onion, chopped
3 tbsp green curry paste
400ml tin coconut milk
360g frozen vegetable mix

600g white fish fillets (such as cod), coarsely chopped
cooked brown rice and lime wedges, to serve (optional)

- Heat the oil in a wok or high-sided frying pan over a high heat. Add the chopped onion and cook for 3–4 minutes, then add the curry paste and cook, stirring, for 1 more minute.
- Pour in the coconut milk and bring to a boil. Reduce the heat to medium-low and add the frozen vegetables and fish.
- Simmer for 15 minutes until the fish is cooked and the vegetables have warmed through. Serve immediately with brown rice and lime wedges, if desired.

Prep	Cook	Kcal	Fats(g)	Carbs(g)	Protein(g)
5 mins	20 mins	351	20	14	29

With brown rice (75g per head):

Prep	Cook	Kcal	Fats(g)	Carbs(g)	Protein(g)
2 mins	20 mins	84	62	17	1.75

Miso Salmon or Tofu with Courgetti Noodles (Serves 2)

Salmon or tofu

2 tbsp miso paste

2 tbsp honey

60ml soy sauce or tamari

2 tbsp grated ginger

2 tbsp apple cider vinegar

1 tbsp sesame oil

2 salmon fillets (about 130g each) or 180g tofu, chopped

2 tsp sesame seeds, to serve

Noodles

400g courgetti noodles

6 radishes, sliced

2 tsp sesame oil

2 tsp ginger, grated

1 tsp honey

2 tbsp soy sauce

juice of 1 lime

- Mix all the salmon or tofu marinade ingredients together. Coat the salmon fillets or chopped tofu in the marinade and refrigerate for at least 20 minutes.
- In the meantime, place the courgetti noodles and sliced radishes in a bowl. Mix all the ingredients for the noodles dressing and pour over the noodles. Mix well and refrigerate.
- Preheat the oven to 180°C (350°F).
- If using salmon, place it in an ovenproof dish and pour some of the marinade over it. Bake for 12 minutes and then turn the grill on for about 2–3 minutes to brown the top. Check often to avoid burning.
- If using tofu, lightly fry and go to the next step.
- Once cooked, serve the salmon or tofu alongside the courgetti noodles. Sprinkle with sesame seeds to serve.

Prep	Cook	Kcal	Fats(g)	Carbs(g)	Protein(g)
20 mins	15 mins	496	30	22	29 (salmon) 17 (tofu)

Creamy Chicken, Mushroom & Spinach Pasta (Serves 3)

. . . .

150g penne

350g skinless chicken breasts

1 tsp plain flour

1 tbsp olive oil

1 tsp dried oregano

1 small onion, diced

2 garlic cloves, sliced

300g mushrooms, sliced

6 sun-dried tomatoes, chopped

125ml plant-based oat cream/ regular cream

300g spinach

basil leaves, to garnish

- Cook the pasta according to the instructions on the packet.
- Chop the chicken fillet, season with salt and pepper and dredge with flour.
- Heat the oil in a large pan and cook the chicken over a medium heat, then season with oregano. Once the chicken is cooked, remove from the pan and set aside.
- In the same pan, sauté the onion and garlic. Next, add the sliced mushrooms and cook for 5–7 minutes until soft and tender. Add the sun-dried tomatoes and cook for another minute.
- Place the cooked chicken back into the pan and add the cream and spinach. Bring to a boil and cook until the spinach has wilted, then season to taste with salt and pepper.
- Add the cooked pasta. Stir well and serve with the basil.

Prep	Cook	Kcal	Fats(g)	Carbs(g)	Protein(g)
10 mins	20 mins	385	14	26	35

Snacks

If you find yourself getting hungry in the afternoon, this might be because you aren't eating enough protein earlier in the day. If you are finding the plan hard, it is fine to have a little something because we want this to be achievable and sustainable. If you are hungry, you are more likely to snack into the evening and make food choices that might not help you feel your best.

The following are some ideas for healthy snacks that will give you a boost of energy without having to resort to sugary snacks.

Protein Balls

• •

handful of almonds
2 tbsp peanut butter
1 tbsp cacao nibs

6–7 Medjool dates
1 tbsp coconut oil

- Blend all the ingredients together in a food processor or high-speed blender, roll into balls and refrigerate.

Note: Keep refrigerated for a slightly chewy texture.

Prep	Cook	Kcal	Fats(g)	Carbs(g)	Protein(g)
10 mins	0 mins	160	11	12	7

Apple & Nut Butter

• •

1 tbsp nut butter
1 apple, sliced

- Spread the nut butter onto slices of apple.

Prep	Cook	Kcal	Fats(g)	Carbs(g)	Protein(g)
5 mins	0 mins	180	18	31	7

Edamame Beans

. . . .

100g frozen edamame beans   sea salt

- These are a great snack and can be bought frozen in bags.
- Once defrosted, warm them up and sprinkle lightly with sea salt.

Prep	Cook	Kcal	Fats(g)	Carbs(g)	Protein(g)
0 mins	0 mins	188	8	13	18

Roasted Chickpeas (Makes about 12 x 30g servings)

. . . .

400g tin chickpeas, rinsed and drained

extra-virgin olive oil, for drizzling

generous pinches of sea salt

paprika, curry powder or other spices (optional)

- Preheat the oven to 220°C (425°F) and line a large baking tray with baking paper.
- Spread the chickpeas on a kitchen towel and pat them dry, removing any loose skins.
- Transfer the dried chickpeas to the baking tray and toss them with a drizzle of olive oil and generous pinches of sea salt.
- Roast the chickpeas for 20–30 minutes, or until golden brown and crisp.
- Remove from the oven and, while the chickpeas are still warm, toss with pinches of your favourite spices.

Note: Store the roasted chickpeas in a loosely covered container at room temperature. They are best eaten within 2 days.

Prep	Cook	Kcal	Fats(g)	Carbs(g)	Protein(g)
5 mins	30 mins	86	2	17	5

Little Treats

Blueberry Protein Ice Cream
• •

145g cottage cheese	4 tbsp dried blueberries
1 banana	75g fresh blueberries
25g Greek yoghurt	

- Place the cottage cheese, banana and yoghurt in a food processor and blend everything together.
- Transfer the mixture into a Tupperware or similar type of container and mix in the dried berries. Cover with a lid and freeze for 45 minutes, then take out of the freezer and mix again. Return the dish to the freezer and chill for a further 45 minutes.
- Take the dish out of the freezer, mix again and serve with fresh berries.

Note: If you keep it in the freezer for longer, then thaw for 10–15 minutes before serving.

Prep	Chill	Kcal	Fats(g)	Carbs(g)	Protein(g)
10 mins	90 mins	243	4	26	28

Matcha Chia Pudding

30g chia seeds
350ml almond milk
2 tsp maple syrup

1 tsp matcha powder
100g fresh or frozen berries,
   to serve

- Mix the chia seeds and almond milk together and place in the fridge. After an hour, mix again and place back in the fridge to chill overnight.
- The next morning, mix in the maple syrup and matcha.
- Divide between two bowls and serve with berries.

Prep	Chill	Kcal	Fats(g)	Carbs(g)	Protein(g)
5 mins	Overnight	275	9	19	23

Green Glow Protein Smoothie

1 small banana
250g spinach
250g kale

1 tbsp almond butter
100ml coconut water
25g cottage cheese

- Place all the ingredients into a high-speed blender and blitz until smooth. Serve immediately.

Prep	Cook	Kcal	Fats(g)	Carbs(g)	Protein(g)
5 mins	0 mins	350	12	34	29

Shopping Lists for the Meal Plans

Cupboard and fridge essentials

Oils and vinegar
Olive oil
Coconut oil
Sesame oil
Balsamic vinegar

Herbs and spices
Ground cinnamon
Ground turmeric
Dried oregano
Chilli flakes

Fruit and vegetables
Onions
Garlic
Lemons and limes

Cupboard
Jasmine rice
Plain flour
Brown rice

Penne (wholemeal preferable)
Rolled oats
Tinned tomatoes
Tinned coconut milk
Tinned chickpeas

Fridge
Greek yoghurt
Plant milk/milk
Eggs

Miscellaneous
Soy sauce or tamari
Tabasco
Chicken stock
Vegetable stock
Bicarbonate of soda
Maple syrup
Honey
Peanut butter

Shopping List for Days 1–7

Fruit and vegetables
2 sweet potatoes
1 cauliflower
Cucumber
Cherry tomatoes
Spring onions

Radishes
Salad leaves
2 medium beetroots
2 bags spinach
900g mushrooms
Mint

Basil
Parsley
Fresh fruit
2 bananas
Frozen blueberries
Frozen vegetable mix

Miscellaneous
Fennel seeds
Chia seeds
Ground almonds
Almond butter
Walnuts
Green curry paste
Yellow curry paste
½ bottle white wine
Miso paste
Dried cranberries

Rice vinegar
2 packets cooked quinoa
Dried red lentils
1 tin pineapple
2 tins kidney beans
Apple cider vinegar

Fridge
1 tub cottage cheese
1 packet feta cheese
400g courgetti noodles

Meat, fish and tofu
400g chicken breasts or tofu
700g skinless chicken breast
8 skinless chicken thighs
4 tins tuna or 400g tofu
2 salmon fillets or 180g tofu
600g white fish fillets

Shopping List for Days 8–14

Fruit and vegetables
530g spinach
1 avocado
3 cauliflowers
140g potatoes
2 (or 4) medium beetroots
4 sweet potatoes
50g courgettes
150g cherry tomatoes
60g rocket
3 shallots
8 radishes
1 cauliflower

Bean sprouts
300g mushrooms
2 large carrots
7 spring onions
Ginger
Basil
Coriander
Dill
2 bananas
Fresh berries
Frozen blueberries
100g frozen strawberries

Miscellaneous
Almond butter
Walnuts
Chia seeds
Ground almonds
Peanuts
Roasted almonds
Nuts and seeds
Roasted peppers
Yellow curry paste
Dried red lentils
Thai red curry paste
Fennel seeds
2 packets cooked quinoa
Spelt flour
4 packets cooked brown rice
Red pesto
Miso paste
2 tins lentils
½ bottle white wine
Sesame seeds

Dried cranberries
Sun-dried tomatoes
Rice vinegar
Apple cider vinegar

Extras
Homemade healthy granola

Fridge
300g cottage cheese
200g (or 400g) feta
50g cottage cheese
8 prosciutto slices
400g courgetti noodles

Meat, fish and tofu
12 skinless chicken thighs
700g skinless chicken breasts
200g salmon or tofu
2 salmon fillets (130g each) or
   180g tofu

Shopping List for Days 15–21

Fruit and vegetables
900g mushrooms
2 bags spinach
2 sweet potatoes
1 cauliflower
Cucumber
Salad leaves
Spinach
2 (or 4) medium beetroots
Cherry tomatoes

6 radishes
Rosemary
Parsley
Mint
Basil
Ginger
2 bananas
Frozen blueberries
Frozen vegetables

Miscellaneous

Chia seeds
Ground almonds
Almond butter
Walnuts
2 tins kidney beans
2 tins pineapple
Raw quinoa
Dijon mustard
Dried red lentils
Rice vinegar
Green curry paste
Yellow curry paste
½ bottle white wine
Fennel seeds
Dried cranberries
Sesame seeds
2 (or 4) packets cooked
  quinoa

Miso paste
Sun-dried tomatoes
Apple cider vinegar

Fridge

Feta
400g courgetti noodles
250ml plant-based oat cream/
  regular cream

Meat, fish and tofu

400g chicken breast or tofu
8 skinless chicken thighs
700g skinless chicken breast
4 tins tuna or 400g tofu
600g white fish fillets (cod)
2 salmon fillets (130g each) or
  180 g tofu

Shopping List for Days 22–30

Fruit and vegetables

2 bags spinach
1 avocado
3 cauliflowers
4 sweet potatoes
50g courgettes
140g potatoes
3 shallots
7 spring onions
Ginger
Bean sprouts
600g mushrooms

4 (or 6) medium beetroots
150g cherry tomatoes
60g rocket
8 radishes
2 large carrots
Dill
Coriander
Basil
2 bananas
Fresh berries
Frozen blueberries
100g frozen strawberries

Miscellaneous
Almond butter
Chia seeds
Fennel seeds
Red pesto
Ground almonds
Walnuts
Peanuts
Roasted almonds
Nuts and seeds
Dried red lentils
Yellow curry paste
4 packets cooked brown rice
Spelt flour
Thick rice noodles
Roasted peppers
Thai red curry paste
4 tins lentils
½ bottle white wine
Sun-dried tomatoes
Sesame seeds

Apple cider vinegar
Miso paste
Dried cranberries
Apple cider vinegar
Rice vinegar

Extras
Homemade healthy granola

Fridge
350g cottage cheese
400g (or 600g) feta
400g courgetti noodles
16 prosciutto slices

Meat, fish and tofu
16 skinless chicken thighs
700g skinless chicken breast
200g salmon or tofu
2 salmon fillets (130g each) or
    180g tofu

WHAT NEXT?

Well done.

What an achievement to have committed to your future health by introducing weights and sticking to the plan. This is only the beginning and I would love for you to think about how you want to keep making change and progress. DON'T STOP NOW.

You should be feeling raring and ready to continue with some of the changes you have made because you feel fitter, calmer and stronger.

The book has armed, empowered and equipped you to understand what it is you need to do. Use this momentum of feeling fitter, calmer and stronger to commit and stick to these lifelong changes you have made over the last 30 days.

Look back and go through your journals so you can see how far you have come. Don't think about how far you may still like to go as this will change your positive mindset.

I have talked about continuing to build strength and this is the perfect opportunity and time to drive forward. Much of what I was wanting you to take away from this is the idea that your body is not seasonal, that doing plans here and there sporadically throughout the year won't benefit you. It will only see you back onto the yoyo pattern many of us find ourselves on, which, as you know, doesn't work.

You now understand the importance of nourishing your body with three wholesome, colourful, protein-rich plates a day. You feel full after each meal and the need for snacking has dissipated. You feel confident in making healthy choices and have adopted a balanced approach. You are no longer self-sabotaging and understand if you go off track for a day this doesn't dictate the rest of the day and equally doesn't mean you have failed.

I realise that you have had to digest a lot of information, but I know that this tried-and-tested approach works and is sustainable and achievable.

This is also the beginning of a wonderful new chapter where you can feel the importance and benefits of adding weights to your life, so you can optimise your wellbeing and build strength from the inside out.

My top tips for you to keep moving forward would be:

- Set SMART goals: specific, measurable, attainable, relevant and timely.

- Keep journalling your progress.

- Keep tracking your symptoms so you can see if there are ever any triggers that make them worse or perhaps anything that really helps you manage them.

- You could repeat the programme. If you did the Beginner's plan, you could move on to the Intermediate plan.

- Join the Owning Your Menopause App to stay accountable and supported and to continue getting fitter, calmer and stronger. (You will get 50 per cent off an annual membership with the code OYMBOOK50).

- Keep your steps up. This is such a big part of continuing your journey forward.

SET S.M.A.R.T GOALS

S.M.A.R.T. is an acronym that guides in the setting of goals and objectives to give better results.

Specific Specific goals are goals that have clear and well-defined objectives.

Measurable Measurable goals mean that you identify exactly what it is you will see, hear and feel when you reach your goal.

Attainable Your goal also needs to be realistic and attainable to be successful. In other words, it should stretch your abilities but still remain possible.

Relevant Your goal should be reasonable, realistic, resourced and results-based.

Timely Every goal needs a target date so that you have a deadline to focus on and something to work towards.

If you start a new plan and realise within a few days you won't be able to sustain it, there's no point in carrying on for another 6 weeks only to revert to your old habits.

You must try to find a sustainable and achievable routine, something you can, and want, to implement for 365 days of the year, not just 6 weeks here and there. I suggest focusing on making small tweaks instead of huge sacrifices or restrictions because the reality is that you won't be able to sustain it.

Goal	Aim	Likely to succeed	Likely to quit
Specific	Make it well-defined so that anyone can understand.	I will do 3 x 30-minute workouts for 1 month, with the intention of building up gradually.	I will do a 30-minute workout every day.
Measurable	How will you know if you have achieved this?	I will plan and make time for these sessions each week and track my improvements in my notebook.	I'll just try to fit it in when I can.
Attainable	Is this something you can do and will have success doing?	I will add some strength sessions each month until I am able to do 3–4 each week. I will start with a comfortable weight and add gradually.	I will get straight into lifting heavy weights 3–4 times a week.
Relevant	Is this something that is important to you?	I would like to future-proof my body for longevity. I want to be fitter, calmer and stronger.	I want to get into shape for . . .
Timely	Will you be able to achieve this in the time frame you have set?	I want to commit to an achievable, sustainable plan that I enjoy for life.	I want to finish this plan and see the results in a month.

Make It Fun

Movement, exercise, fitness – whatever you would like to call it – needs to be enjoyable and fun in order to make it stick and for you to start. We want to get to a place where it is not a chore and something we feel we have to do, but rather something that we want to do because it is a pleasurable addition to our lifestyle choices.

Invite a friend or colleague to join you because starting and sticking to something with a friend in tow is always a lot more fun and you can champion and encourage each other to keep going on the harder days.

Try new things – don't think you can only do one type of exercise class. As we have seen in Chapter 8, there are many different ways to move. Make the time to try and find something that will be worthwhile.

Plan

Planning the week and how it will look can be helpful in committing and sticking to a plan and holding yourself accountable. Most of us know what is coming up, and we can sit and think, 'Okay, this is how my week will look.' This way, you can potentially avoid the self-sabotage that so many of us find ourselves doing.

Every Sunday, sit down and plan out your week. Think about the exercise you are going to do and the meals you will be eating to nourish your body and try to stick with it – life can get in the way, and that's okay, but having a plan and deviating occasionally is better than no plan at all.

Long-term Changes

If you want to get yourself to a place where you can do this, you need to accept this is a lifestyle choice that you must implement all year round. Some of you might be bored with the yoyoing diet world you find yourself in and the thought of breaking this cycle is something you've wanted to do for years – well, this is your opportunity.

You can't put a time limit on your health. There should ultimately never be an end goal. Optimising your future health is a never-ending journey to be enjoyed and be grateful for.

ACKNOWLEDGEMENTS

I thank my amazingly patient and incredible children: Oliver, Sophie and Rupert.

I appreciate all of your support while I've been working on this book. It hasn't been easy, but none of you have complained, which means a lot to me. Sophie, I wrote a lot of this with you in mind, so I hope it helps make your future easier. Ollie and Rupert, I wrote this so you can be great future partners, friends and colleagues. And to all of you, remember that even if your voice is small, you can still have an impact on others and help make a difference.

To my mum, I know you are amazed that I have written a book considering my track record at school. This only highlights my message that it's never too late to change and that you cannot let your past determine your future. Always try and do something you'd been convinced you couldn't achieve. Constantly challenge yourself regardless.

To my darling Daddy, who would have been so proud (and shocked?). It saddens me that I never got to tell you I was writing a book, but I know you have sat with me as I typed away endlessly, questioning myself at times and encouraging me to keep at it when I was questioning myself. You taught me that nothing is impossible, and we must honestly believe in ourselves and show what we are capable of.

And to my gorgeous sister, Georgia, thank you for your encouragement from afar in Kenya and for offering your services and many suggestions. Given you are an English scholar, I was terrified to share it with you until I reached the end, but your unwavering support has meant the world to me.

To my lovely friends, who I have barely seen – thank you for your patience and support. You all know how passionate I am about helping women thrive, and I have loved that you have often turned to me as a source of information. Many of you have raised eyebrows when I suggested you may be in perimenopause. Occasionally, I've probably been the most annoying guest at a dinner party, talking about menopause.

To my lovely Swiss ladies, I know that will resonate with you as on our recent trip you called me a M~~enopa~~ ~~sa~~id with love, I know. Thank you all for believing in me and always championing me when I need it most.

Thank you also to the fantastic ladies who contribute to the platform Owning Your Menopause. I know you are as passionate about helping women as I am, and I thank you for being a part of the platform.

I never thought I would say thank you to social media, but Instagram has given me a substantial reach and enabled me to help so many women. It allowed me to realise what I needed to create to support other women. Thank you to everyone who has followed me. You have given me the strength to carry on when I felt unsure about what I was doing. Social media is a scary, daunting place for a woman going through menopause and midlife.

Thank you to all those who have subscribed to Owning Your Menopause. It is an absolute pleasure to get up and work out with you every day and see your lovely faces smiling back. You are all committed, and I hope you continue your journey with us, always building strength and future-proofing your body.

Nicky Ross, my editor, well, what do I say? When I got your email at the end of January 2023, it was as if all my dreams had come true. I had been penning something for around 6 months, as writing a book was a dream I didn't know how to fulfil, mostly because of time constraints but also because I lacked confidence.

However, as soon as I spoke to you, I knew we had something. You understood me, my message and what I desperately wanted to share to help other women. You let my brain jump around and spill out onto the paper with little structure, but you knew how to guide me to settle into it, find order, and just go for it.

Nicola Way, who would have ever thought we would work together? I know you had every intention of taking time out after leaving your previous job, but I think the temptation of supporting your friend with the tasks she continued to set herself was too great for you to sit back and watch. And I am so grateful you didn't. I would be absolutely out of my depth. Your belief in what I am doing has been instrumental when I have felt over my head.

Last but not least, my incredibly supportive husband, Gerry. I know this has not been easy on us and, at times, we both felt I'd taken on too much. We both know how stubborn I am and that I had been talking about writing a book for some time. So, when I was approached, the opportunity was too good to say no. Thank you for holding the fort on the weekends that I have locked myself away.

ABOUT THE AUTHOR

Kate Rowe-Ham is a Women's Health Coach with a special interest in menopause fitness and nutrition, and the founder of Owning Your Menopause.

Kate is passionate about educating women on how to exercise and nourish their bodies at this time. She wants to educate women on the benefits of movement and diet, so they can see how these play a fundamental role in managing many of the symptoms associated with menopause.

Qualifying as a Level 3 Personal Trainer later in life, alongside raising her three children and experiencing her own issues with perimenopause, has given Kate a unique insight into how isolating this journey can be. It is well noted that in midlife, a woman's needs fall by the wayside as we often juggle many balls. Kate knows first-hand that the debilitating effects of menopause can leave women feeling overwhelmed, invisible and anxious. She is on a mission to empower and educate to allow women to see that this can be a time to thrive.

As a trusted expert in her field, Kate has become a 'go-to' Personal Trainer known for her specialised approach to ensuring women get the correct evidence-based information on how to train effectively and nourish their bodies through menopause. She believes that so many women miss out on optimising their midlife and menopause experience due to not understanding how to adapt their lifestyle during this phase.

Kate is encouraging women to reframe their mindset from always seeing movement as a punishment and aiming for the aesthetic benefits to educating women to appreciate the benefits exercise has on their heart, bones, joints, muscles, brain and mental health.

Over the years, Kate has worked with well-known brands, such as Sweaty Betty, Nike, Lucozade Sport, Fatface and JD Williams. She has been featured in several press articles and publications, including *The Times*, *Women's Health*, *Fit & Well*, *Women's Fitness*, *Prima*, *Liz Earle Wellbeing*, *Good Housekeeping*, *Woman & Home* and *Coach*. She has also been a podcast guest with *Wild Nutrition*, *Creative Impact*, This Is Nessie, Sober Dave, Lawrence Price, and Gaby Logan's *The Mid Point* and has appeared on Channel 4's *Sunday Brunch* and BBC News. Currently, Kate is the Energy Field Director at Big Retreat Wales, and one of her favourite things is to speak at wellness events across the country to empower women to own their menopause.

Recognising that there has been a lack of support and education for women in this demographic led Kate to spearhead the creation of the Owning Your Menopause app. This offering provides a platform that reshapes what training means to women going through menopause. Through in-depth research, self-testing, coaching and refinement, Kate is providing women with much-needed information and support. She would love every woman to know that they have the potential to be strong in mind and body regardless of their starting point and that with the right support, they can embrace menopause and midlife. Kate aims to help women find a path to a healthier lifestyle, giving them the tools they need to adopt a sustainable approach to exercise.

Instagram: https://www.instagram.com/katerh_fitness/
Website: www.katerhfitness.com
Email: kate@owningyourmenopause.com

ENDNOTES

1. https://www.msdmanuals.com/en-au/home/women-s-health-issues/biology-of-the-female-reproductive-system/menstrual-cycle/
2. https://pubmed.ncbi.nlm.nih.gov/951489/
3. https://www.forthwithlife.co.uk/blog/menopause-hormones/
4. https://www.fawcettsociety.org.uk/news/landmark-study-menopausal-women-let-down-by-employers-and-healthcare-providers/
5. https://pubmed.ncbi.nlm.nih.gov/36675477/
6 https://www.webmd.com/women/estrogen-and-womens-emotions
7. https://pubmed.ncbi.nlm.nih.gov/21961723/
8. https://menopausecare.co.uk/body-identical-hrt/
9. https://www.ncbi.nlm.nih.gov/pmc/articles/PMC1158967/
10. https://www.endocrine.org/patient-engagement/endocrine-library/menopause-and-bone-loss
11. https://www.endocrine.org/patient-engagement/endocrine-library/menopause-and-bone-loss
12. https://www.nhs.uk/conditions/dexa-scan/
13. https://patient.info/doctor/frax-fracture-risk-assessment-tool
14. https://www.ncbi.nlm.nih.gov/pmc/articles/PMC2804956/
15. https://www.nhs.uk/live-well/exercise/exercise-guidelines/physical-activity-guidelines-for-adults-aged-19-to-64/
16. https://academic.oup.com/eurjpc/advance-article/doi/10.1093/eurjpc/zwad229/7226309
17. https://www.news-medical.net/health/How-Does-Menopause-Affect-the-Brain.aspx
18. https://publications.parliament.uk/pa/cm5803/cmselect/cmwomeq/91/report.html

19. https://www.sleepfoundation.org/physical-activity/exercise-and-sleep
20. https://www.cancerresearchuk.org/about-cancer/causes-of-cancer/bodyweight-and-cancer/how-does-obesity-cause-cancer
21. https://www.ons.gov.uk/peoplepopulationandcommunity/birthsdeathsandmarriages/lifeexpectancies/articles/howhaslifeexpectancychangedovertime/2015-09-09
22. https://www.nhs.uk/live-well/exercise/exercise-guidelines/physical-activity-guidelines-for-adults-aged-19-to-64/
23. https://www.cdc.gov/physicalactivity/index.html
24. https://www.builtlean.com/muscles-grow/
25. https://www.unm.edu/~lkravitz/Article%20folder/musclesgrowLK.html
26. https://www.nhs.uk/live-well/exercise/running-and-aerobic-exercises/walking-for-health/
27. https://steelfitusa.com/blogs/health-and-wellness/calculate-tdee
28. https://www.verywellfit.com/thermic-effect-of-food-1231350
29. https://www.thehealthylivingcentre.co.uk/contents/downloads/REPs_Members_PAR_questionnaire.pdf
30. https://www.mayoclinic.org/healthy-lifestyle/fitness/in-depth/core-exercises/art-20044751
31. https://www.shape.com/fitness/tips/3-things-you-need-do-immediately-after-workout
32. https://www.healthline.com/health/exercise-fitness/rest-day#signs-you-need-rest
33. https://www.verywellfit.com/do-athletes-need-extra-sleep-3120087
34. https://www.thensf.org/
35. https://www.theinsomniaclinic.co.uk/blog//how-to-improve-sleep-during-the-menopause
36. https://www.verywellfit.com/after-exercise-does-an-ice-water-bath-speed-recovery-3120571
37. https://casereports.bmj.com/content/2018/bcr-2018-225007
38. https://www.ncbi.nlm.nih.gov/pmc/articles/PMC5810528

39. https://my.clevelandclinic.org/health/body/22804-ghrelin
40. https://www.news-medical.net/health/Ghrelin-and-Sleep.aspx
41. https://www.diabetes.org.uk/guide-to-diabetes/life-with-diabetes/menopause
42. https://patient.info/news-and-features/whats-the-recommended-calorie-intake-for-women.
43. https://www.ncbi.nlm.nih.gov/pmc/articles/PMC6390141/
44. https://pubmed.ncbi.nlm.nih.gov/29673827/
45. https://www.health.harvard.edu/womens-health/why-does-alcohol-affect-women-differently
46. https://www.healthcentral.com/condition/menopause/menopause-alcohol

INDEX

Note: page numbers in **bold** refer to diagrams.